PROGRESS AND PROBLEMS IN MEDICAL AND DENTAL EDUCATION

Federal Support Versus Federal Control

A REPORT OF THE CARNEGIE COUNCIL
ON POLICY STUDIES IN HIGHER EDUCATION

*A report of the
Carnegie Council
on Policy Studies
in Higher Education*

PROGRESS AND PROBLEMS IN MEDICAL AND DENTAL EDUCATION

Federal Support Versus
Federal Control

Jossey-Bass Publishers
San Francisco · Washington · London · 1976

PROGRESS AND PROBLEMS IN MEDICAL AND DENTAL EDUCATION
Federal Support Versus Federal Control
The Carnegie Council on Policy Studies in Higher Education

Copyright © 1976 by: The Carnegie Foundation
                       for the Advancement of Teaching

                       Jossey-Bass, Inc., Publishers
                       615 Montgomery Street
                       San Francisco, California 94111

                       Jossey-Bass Limited
                       44 Hatton Garden
                       London EC1N 8ER

*This report is issued by the Carnegie Council on Policy Studies
in Higher Education with headquarters at 2150 Shattuck Avenue,
Berkeley, California 94704.*

*Copies are available from Jossey-Bass, San Francisco,
for the United States, Canada, and Possessions.
Copies for the rest of the world are available from
Jossey-Bass, London.*

Library of Congress Catalogue Card Number LC 76-11964

International Standard Book Number ISBN 0-87589-295-7

Manufactured in the United States of America

DESIGN BY WILLI BAUM

FIRST EDITION

Code 7615

The Carnegie Council Series

The Federal Role in Postsecondary
Education: Unfinished Business,
1975-1980
*The Carnegie Council on Policy
Studies in Higher Education*

More than Survival: Prospects
for Higher Education in a
Period of Uncertainty
*The Carnegie Foundation for
the Advancement of Teaching*

Making Affirmative Action Work
in Higher Education: An Analysis
of Institutional and Federal
Policies with Recommendations
*The Carnegie Council on Policy
Studies in Higher Education*

Presidents Confront Reality:
From Edifice Complex to
University Without Walls
*Lyman A. Glenny, John R. Shea,
Janet H. Ruyle, Kathryn H. Freschi*

Low or No Tuition: The Feasibil-
ity of a National Policy for the
First Two Years of College
*The Carnegie Council on Policy
Studies in Higher Education*

Managing Multicampus Systems:
Effective Administration in an
Unsteady State
Eugene C. Lee, Frank M. Bowen

Challenges Past, Challenges
Present: An Analysis of
American Higher Education
Since 1930
David D. Henry

The States and Higher
Education: A Proud Past
and a Vital Future
*The Carnegie Foundation for
the Advancement of Teaching*

Progress and Problems in Medical
and Dental Education: Federal
Support Versus Federal Control
*The Carnegie Council on Policy
Studies in Higher Education*

Contents

Preface

The Carnegie Council on Policy Studies in Higher Education has a special and continuing interest in health-manpower education. Our interest is the legacy of a long tradition. The famous Flexner report of 1910, which specified the model of the modern science- and research-oriented medical school, was sponsored by The Carnegie Foundation for the Advancement of Teaching. Over the years, the Carnegie Corporation of New York and the Carnegie Foundation have provided support for many improvements and innovations in medical and dental education.

Early in its history, the Carnegie Commission on Higher Education (predecessor of the Carnegie Council) selected medical and dental education as an area of special concern in higher education to which it would devote one of its special reports. That report, *Higher Education and the Nation's Health,* issued in the fall of 1970, proved to be one of the most influential of the Commission's 22 special reports. Many of the most significant features of the Comprehensive Health Manpower Act of 1971 were strongly influenced by it. These included:

- The principle of providing a basic and continuing federal floor of support for medical and dental schools in the form of capitation (per student) payments.
- The provision of bonuses to the schools for expansion of places and acceleration of programs.
- The provision of federal funds for curriculum reform and innovation.

- Federal funds for an adequate program of student grants and loans.
- Federal support for the training of physician's and dental assistants.
- Creation of a national health service corps.[1]
- Federal funds for construction and start-up grants for new medical and dental schools. (The Commission warned, however, that too many communities were seeking to establish new medical schools and that only nine new schools were needed to achieve adequate geographic distribution.)
- Federal funds to support the development of area health education centers, which would be affiliated with university health science centers and would perform all the functions of those centers except for the basic education of M.D. and D.D.S. candidates. The area health education centers, for which the Commission suggested 126 geographically distributed locations, would improve the quality of health training and health care in their areas, help to overcome problems of geographic maldistribution of health manpower, and remove the pressure in many communities for the establishment of new medical schools.

Under the impetus of the 1971 legislation, much has been accomplished. In fact, many of the needed changes were under way before that legislation was enacted. The record of expansion of medical and dental education, of curriculum reform, of decentralization of clinical training, and—very recently—of a reversal of the longtime trend toward excessive specialization in medical education is remarkable. Yet many of the problems remain—too much reliance on foreign medical graduates, little or no progress in overcoming geographic maldistribution of health manpower, and, as yet, too little impact of shifting patterns of medical training on overspecialization in medical practice.

The Congress is understandably concerned over these problems but, in its anxiety to combat them, is considering legislative

---

[1]This was actually created under separate legislation adopted by Congress toward the end of 1970.

provisions that would saddle the university health science centers with a set of complex and cumbersome federal controls. This report urges a policy of sustained and consistent federal support of medical and dental education, along with the provision of strong incentives toward needed changes, rather than excessive controls. It is a report in the tradition of the Carnegie Commission's 1970 report, but with central orientation toward the more complex legislative issues that have emerged in the last six years. Like that report, it is focused on medical and dental education, rather than on the broader subject of all health-manpower education. This is because there are special controversies that have arisen over federal policies toward the training of physicians and dentists that are not present in the training of other health manpower.

The Council wishes to express its appreciation for the useful comments and suggestions of those who read an earlier draft of this report. They include: Dr. John A. D. Cooper, president, Association of American Medical Colleges; Dr. Robert Ebert, dean, Harvard Medical School; Dr. Thomas Ginley, secretary, Council on Dental Education, American Dental Association; Dr. Charles V. Kidd, executive secretary, Association of American Universities; Dr. Philip R. Lee, director, Health Policy Program, School of Medicine, University of California, San Francisco; Dr. Robert Q. Marston, president, University of Florida; Dr. Dale Redig, dean, School of Dentistry, University of the Pacific; Dr. Sheldon Rovin, dean, School of Dentistry, University of Washington; and Dr. C. H. W. Ruhe, director, Division of Medical Education, American Medical Association.

We also wish to express our thanks to the members of our staff who contributed to the work of this report, especially Dr. Margaret S. Gordon, who was assisted by Ruth Goto and Stanley Severson.

William G. Bowen
President
Princeton University

Ernest L. Boyer
Chancellor
State University of New York

Nolen Ellison
President
Cuyahoga Community College

E. K. Fretwell, Jr.
President
State University of New York College at Buffalo

Margaret L. A. MacVicar
Associate Professor of Physics
Massachusetts Institute of Technology

Rosemary Park
Professor of Education Emeritus
University of California, Los Angeles

James A. Perkins
Chairman of the Board
International Council for Educational Development

Alan Pifer, *ex officio*
President
The Carnegie Foundation for the Advancement of Teaching

Joseph B. Platt
President
Harvey Mudd College

Lois Rice
Vice-President
College Entrance Examination Board

William M. Roth
Regent of the University of California

Pauline Tompkins
President
Cedar Crest College

William Van Alstyne
Professor of Law
Duke University

Clark Kerr
Chairperson
Carnegie Council on Policy Studies in Higher Education

PROGRESS AND PROBLEMS IN MEDICAL AND DENTAL EDUCATION

Federal Support
Versus
Federal Control

A REPORT OF THE CARNEGIE COUNCIL
ON POLICY STUDIES IN HIGHER EDUCATION

1

Three Warnings
and Five Urgent
Recommendations

In the spring of 1970, an official estimate that there was a shortage of 50,000 physicians in the United States was widely quoted. But between 1970 and the end of 1975, the total number of active physicians and osteopaths rose from about 323,000 to an estimated 378,000, or by about 55,000.

Does this remarkable increase mean that the shortage has disappeared? One can get a variety of answers to this question, depending on the perspectives of those replying. Some warn of an impending, if not an actual, surplus. Some say that the increase in overall supply has not helped to overcome geographic disparities in supply, which in fact are worsening. Many argue that, despite the increase in supply, we are plagued by a surplus of specialists and a shortage of primary-care physicians.

One aspect of this situation, however, has received surprisingly little attention from the professional associations particularly concerned with health manpower. In the face of rapid increases in the supply of physicians graduating from existing schools, we are in serious danger of developing too many medical schools. On the whole, the chief reason for new medical schools now is to achieve a more adequate geographic distribution of schools, for there is abundant evidence that the existence of a medical school in a community contributes to increasing the supply of health manpower and can make an important contribution to improving the quality of available medical care. There may also be a case for a few medical-education programs designed specifically to encourage members of minority groups to train for the medical profession.

In addition to the 114 medical schools that now enroll students, there are at least 13 additional schools in various stages of development and many more that are being proposed in various communities. We believe that most of these developing schools are unnecessary. Failure to impose stricter controls by combined federal and state action over the development of new medical schools could well contribute to an excessive increase in the supply of physicians—and at very great cost, because the expenditures associated with development of a new medical school are heavy. Among the measures urgently needed is greater centralization of control within the federal government for approval of start-up and construction funds for new medical schools, and discontinuation of the authorization of the Veterans Administration to provide funds for new schools.

We believe that there is a clear case for a new medical school in one community—Wilmington, Delaware—that has no established or developing school. Unlike most of the other states that lack a medical school, Delaware is highly urbanized, and the case for a university health science center in Wilmington is strong. Arizona and Florida are rapidly growing states, each of which may eventually need an additional medical school.

There are only 59 dental schools, compared with the 114 existing medical schools, but the dentist-population ratio has always been far below the physician-population ratio, and this will probably continue to be true. The size of some of the existing dental schools needs to be increased. Arizona needs a dental school (it now has none), and an additional dental school will probably be needed in Florida, which has only one recently developed school.[1]

---

[1] For more detailed discussion, see Section 6.

First Warning: *We are in serious danger of developing too many new medical schools, and decisive steps need to be taken by both federal and state governments to stop this trend.*

We recommend only one new medical school in a community that now has no existing or developing school—Wilmington, Delaware. We also see a need for one new dental school in Arizona.

We share the views of those who believe that the critical needs now are to overcome geographic maldistribution of health manpower and to increase the proportion of physicians who are engaged in primary care. But we strongly believe that the primary emphasis should be on creating incentives to attract health professionals to underserved areas and to encourage training programs for primary-care physicians, rather than to impose rigid federal controls on medical and dental education.

Many of the legislative proposals that have been under serious consideration by Congress in the last few years have involved the imposition of stringent, and sometimes unwieldy, federal controls. These have included: (1) capitation payback requirements for students who do not practice in underserved areas following graduation; (2) provisions requiring schools, as a condition of their receiving capitation payments, to include in their classes a certain proportion of students who hold National Health Service Corps scholarships; (3) provisions requiring schools, as a condition of their receiving capitation payments, to provide all M.D. and D.D.S. candidates with at least six weeks of training in a setting remote from the main teaching facility of the school; and (4) a variety of provisions establishing strict federal controls over graduate residency programs.

Granted the seriousness of the problems that these proposals are designed to meet, we do not believe that strict federal controls represent the best way of meeting them. They would involve unwarranted interference with academic decisions of the schools and a degree of federal control over the allocation of health manpower that goes far beyond interference in any other field. While favoring federal intervention to achieve desirable social objectives, we share the growing national concern over the size of the federal bureaucracy and its unwieldy powers. Perhaps even more important, rigid controls over the allocation of manpower tend to give rise to evasions that exacerbate the complexity of administrative control.

We also believe that more progress has been made toward reform in medical and dental education than proponents of stringent controls are prepared to admit and that these reforms are likely to lead to an increased emphasis on primary care and a willingness to serve in underserved areas, beyond any results that are as yet statistically measurable. Among these developments are:

- Widespread curriculum reform in medical schools and, to some extent, in dental schools, emphasizing in particular early exposure of the student to clinical experience and a much more conscious effort to relate basic science training to clinical training
- Considerable progress in accelerating medical and dental education
- Involvement of a number of schools in programs to improve the quality of health care in their communities and to increase access to prepaid health care
- Substantial progress toward the decentralization of medical and dental education through the development of area health education centers and other types of decentralized clinical-training programs
- Impressive increases in the enrollment of women and members of minority groups in both medical and dental schools
- A substantial shift—not apparent until the last few years—toward primary care and away from specialization in first-year medical residencies

We urge, and we propose, the provision of financial incentives to medical and dental schools to continue these trends, rather than the subjection of these branches of higher education to unparalleled federal controls.

Figure 1 highlights the type of innovative changes that have received increasing emphasis in university health science centers. In addition, special mention needs to be made of the development of the National Health Service Corps (NHSC) and the associated NHSC scholarship program. The foundations of the expanded NHSC program now contemplated by Congress have been successfully laid.

Figure 1. Innovative changes in university health science centers

Emphasis on Primary Care

Decentralized Clinical Education and Area Health Education Centers

Curriculum Reform

Accelerated Education Programs

Physician's Assistant and Dental Auxiliary Programs

Special Emphasis on Recruitment of Minorities

Involvement in Community Prepaid Health Care Plans

Special Two-Year Medical Education Program for Ph.D.'s

Cooperation with Agricultural Extension

Second Warning: *There is a critical danger that concern over geographic maldistribution of health manpower and overspecialization in medicine will lead to excessive and unwieldy federal controls rather than to policies emphasizing incentives to effect the required changes.*[2]

In the last few decades, we have become far too dependent on an inflow of foreign medical graduates (FMGs) in meeting our physician-supply problems. By the early 1970s about one-fifth of all practicing physicians and nearly one-third of those in internships and residencies were FMGs. But in view of the rapid increase that is now taking place in the number of U.S. medical graduates, a continued heavy inflow of FMGs could greatly exacerbate the dimensions of a possible future surplus. Our projections, which assume a gradual decline in the inflow of FMGs, indicate that the ratio of physicians to population will reach an unprecedented level by the mid-1980s (Figure 2).

Thus, we believe that the measures now under consideration to discontinue preferential immigration status for FMGs and to require them to meet the same standards as U.S. medical graduates before entering residency training or medical practice should be promptly adopted. We would not deny qualified FMGs the right to pursue graduate medical education in the United States on a visiting-scholar basis, but we look forward to the time when the United States will contribute to raising the quality of health care in underdeveloped countries by exporting U.S.-trained physicians rather than depending on foreign countries for its supply.

The issue of the supply of dentists has not been debated as vigorously as the question of physician supply. There has been less evidence of a shortage of dentists and almost no influx of foreign-trained dentists. The demand for dental care has been rising under the impact of rapidly spreading insurance coverage for dental care, but so has the number of U.S. dental graduates. Although the trend toward increasing insurance coverage is certain to continue until the extent of protection for dental care

[2] For more detailed discussion, see Section 4.

Figure 2. Active physicians[a] and dentists per 100,000 population, actual, 1930 to 1970, and projected, 1975 to 1990

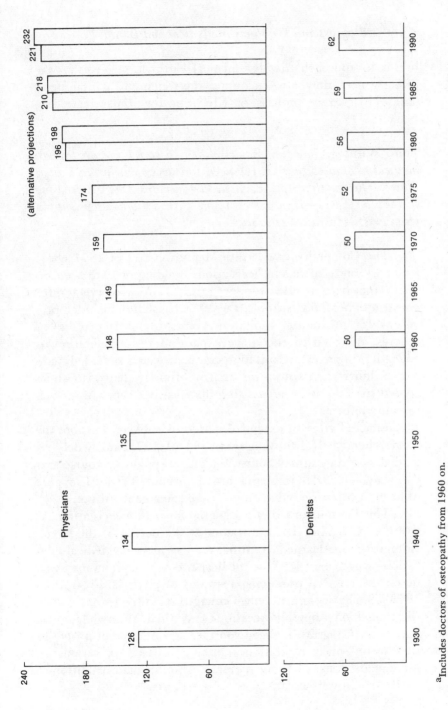

[a]Includes doctors of osteopathy from 1960 on.

Sources: Fein (1967); U.S. Bureau of the Census (annual); U.S. Public Health Service (1974); and Carnegie Council projections of physicians.

begins to approach that for medical care, we believe that the primary need now is to encourage the training of dental auxiliaries and greater emphasis on education for primary-care dentistry.

Third Warning: *The time has come to cease relying on foreign medical graduates to meet the need for physicians in the United States. The number of U.S. medical graduates is now increasing so rapidly that we can expect ample future increases in supply from existing medical schools.*[3]

The Comprehensive Health Manpower Act of 1971 was a landmark piece of federal legislation. Building on earlier enactments that had provided support primarily for research and for construction of new schools, the 1971 legislation included provisions for substantial capitation grants to health-professions schools, designed to encourage expansion and acceleration of education programs. (Capitation grants provide a specified number of dollars to a school for each full-time student.) It also included special-project grants to induce various types of innovation and reform.

Enacted after an extended period of public discussion, the Comprehensive Health Manpower Act of 1971 was widely regarded as setting a new course for federal policy—a course that was expected to determine the broad outlines of federal support of health professions education for the foreseeable future.

This has not turned out to be the fate of the legislation. As early as November 1973, a leading spokesperson of the Nixon Administration warned of cutbacks in support of medical education, suggesting that "the medical education system may well be on the verge of producing a surplus of physicians" (Boffey, 1973). Similar comments have emerged from the federal executive branch on numerous occasions since then. Meanwhile, as we have seen, Congress has been considering a number of proposals that would make capitation grants conditional on various requirements designed to overcome geographic maldistribution of health manpower and an excess of specialists.

[3]For more detailed discussion, see Section 4.

We believe that the federal government should provide a basic floor of support to university health science centers that is not dependent on evidence of shortages and that is contingent only on reasonable requirements calling for maintenance of enrollment and of expenditures from nonfederal sources.

University health science centers are a national resource. They provide substantial social benefits over and above the individual pecuniary benefits that flow to their graduates. The nation has an important stake in continued progress toward combating disease and in maintaining high standards of health among its residents.

In addition, physicians and, though to a considerably lesser extent, dentists are highly mobile geographically. A majority of physicians do not practice in the states in which they received their M.D. degrees. Thus, although many of the states have an excellent record of support to medical and dental education, and although such support has increased substantially in recent years, the record of the states is very uneven and there is no clearcut relationship between a state's investment in medical and dental education and its supply of physicians and dentists.

This means that the federal government has an important responsibility for the national supply of physicians and dentists. In recognition of this responsibility and of the social benefits that flow from medical and dental education, it should provide a basic floor of support that represents a stable but modest proportion of educational costs per student. Once a school is assured that this basic federal support will be forthcoming year after year on a stable basis, it can then seek supplementary support from other public (chiefly state) and private sources. This approach is far preferable to the provision of "financial distress" grants—a practice that developed in the late 1960s—which are designed to "bail a school out" of its financial difficulties and which thus provide a disincentive to the provision of support from nonfederal sources.

Urgent recommendation 1: *The nation has a vital stake in maintaining high standards of health among its residents. In recognition of the social benefits flowing from medical and dental education, the federal government should pursue a stable policy* *of financial support of university health science centers. It should provide a basic floor of support for these centers which can be supplemented by support from state governments and private sources.*[4]

The problem of geographic maldistribution of health manpower is serious. Particularly deficient in manpower are states with low per capita income, rural areas generally, and inner-city areas. The more affluent portions of cities and suburban areas tend to be more adequately supplied and are sometimes oversupplied with physicians, dentists, and other health professionals.

This problem is not unique to the United States. It is found in every industrial country and is explained by the natural desire of health professionals for the higher incomes that are associated with urban practice and for the social amenities of urban life for themselves and their families. It is a problem not easily overcome. In fact, some medical economists, for example, Fuchs (1974), believe it cannot be overcome.

Our view is that geographic maldistribution of health manpower can be substantially alleviated, but only through a combination of policies that create stronger incentives for health professionals to practice in underserved areas. These policies include: (1) expansion of the National Health Service Corps and the associated National Health Service Corps scholarship program; (2) improved financing of medical care, including financial incentives for practicing in underserved areas; (3) changes in reimbursement policies under such federal programs as Medicare and Medicaid, which now encourage subspecialization and do not provide adequately for primary care; (4) continued development and expansion of area health education centers; and (5) continued development and expansion of physician's assistant, nurse practitioner, and dental auxiliary programs, along with improvements in state licensing provisions and with emphasis on educational approaches (such as preceptorships) that will encourage these physician and dentist extenders to serve in underserved areas.

[4]For more detailed discussion, see Sections 3 and 4.

Fortunately, these policies tend to reinforce one another. For example, area health education centers provide appropriate environments for a considerable part of the clinical training of primary-care physicians, dentists, and other health personnel. They also provide a good setting for at least part of the training of physician and dentist extenders.

We believe that health manpower legislation should include provisions—which we spell out more fully in later sections—designed to encourage all these developments without imposing unreasonable requirements on university health science centers or on their students. Although we have mentioned improved financing of medical care, we shall not consider this issue in detail, because it goes beyond the terms of reference of the Carnegie Council, which is concerned with higher education.

In reviewing the developments of the last decade, we are impressed with the considerable progress several states have made toward decentralizing medical and dental education, on their own initiative or with a combination of state and federal funds. We believe that there should be a more consciously developed federal-state partnership toward overcoming geographic disparities in health manpower, as well as more effective coordination of the various federal programs involved with these problems. We spell out our suggestions in greater detail in later sections of this report.[5]

Urgent recommendation 2: *The geographic disparities in the supply of health manpower will be overcome only with great difficulty and through a combination of policies that provide positive incentives for physicians, dentists, and other health professionals to practice in underserved areas. There should be more effective coordination among existing federal programs and greater emphasis on federal-state cooperation in overcoming geographic maldistribution.*

The trend toward excessive specialization in the medical profession has led to an excess supply of specialists, especially

---

[5] For more detailed discussion, see Sections 3, 4, 5, 7, and 8.

of surgeons, in many parts of the country and a deficiency of primary-care physicians. This problem is also of growing concern in dentistry.

Just in the last few years, however, the proportion of first-year medical residents entering primary-care training has increased impressively. A combination of factors, including federal capitation payments for residents in primary-care training, is probably responsible. The progress that is being made suggests the desirability of continuing policies that provide inducements toward greater emphasis on primary-care training, rather than rigid federal controls. The problem cannot be separated from the problem of geographic maldistribution, because such developments as decentralized clinical training for M.D. candidates and residents create a favorable environment for primary-care training.

Urgent recommendation 3: *The federal government should continue to provide incentives for both students and schools to emphasize primary-care training, rather than establish complex federal controls.*[6]

There is a grave danger that recent attacks on the advancement of knowledge in modern medicine—notably that of Illich (1976)—may lead to a decline in federal support of medical research. A stable federal policy of research support is vital to continued progress in combating disease. The importance of such a policy has recently been emphasized by the report of the President's Biomedical Research Panel:

> The United States can take pride in a remarkably productive biomedical and behavioral research effort. The Panel is convinced that despite the appearance of strains in the structure and some dislocation in the parts, the edifice is sound. No testimony is more eloquent than that found in the reports of the eleven interdisciplinary groups made up of 160 of the most

---

[6] For more detailed discussion, see Section 4.

distinguished scientists in the United States enlisted by the Panel to assess the current state of biomedical and behavioral science. Readers of these unique and remarkable reports . . . will sense the restrained elation of the authors, who tell us that the successes of the last three decades portend an acceleration in the pace of discovery in the immediate and the distant future. The remarkable science base of our nation, built so painstakingly and evaluated with such optimism by the interdisciplinary groups, is an indispensable national resource; this science base provides the only sound basis for learning how to prevent and control diseases [U.S. Department of Health, Education, and Welfare, 1976b, p. 1].

The research capabilities of university health science centers cannot be maintained in the face of "stop and go" federal support. In fact, university health science centers experienced more pronounced increases in research support in the early 1970s than did higher education as a whole, but this advantage disappeared between fiscal 1974 and 1975, when research funds allocated to medical schools fell sharply in constant dollars. We believe that federal funds for research in the health field should increase at least as rapidly as the gross national product, and perhaps even more rapidly in the coming years.

At the same time, we agree with a number of medical experts that research oriented to the development of more and more complex technologies has been overemphasized. We need to support research on methods of achieving greater efficiency in health-manpower education and in the delivery of health care as well as biomedical research. And, along with the President's Biomedical Research Panel, we urge that federal research allocations cover the full costs of research projects, including indirect costs. Present requirements for institutional contributions frequently result in a diversion of funds from instructional and other expenditures.[7]

[7] See the recommendation of the Carnegie Commission (1970, p. 73).

Urgent recommendation 4: *The federal government should pursue a stable and consistent policy of support of research in the health sciences, increasing its allocations for this purpose along with the rise in real GNP. Federal allocations should cover full research costs and should encourage increased emphasis on ways of achieving greater efficiency in the training of health manpower and in the delivery of health care.*

Finally, we believe that there must be greatly increased emphasis on health education in our society. There is much evidence that the comparatively high mortality rates for males in the United States from middle age onward are associated with unwise diets, excessive smoking, use of alcohol and drugs, and accidents.[8] Advancement in the health sciences can do little to combat these problems, although it can often prolong the lives of the victims.

Dental educators also point out that the elimination or reduction of smoking and drinking would virtually eliminate oral cancer.

Under the impact of the regional medical programs and subsequent health planning legislation,[9] there has, in fact, been substantial development of programs of health education at the regional and local level. This effort should be continued, and the future should see an increasing emphasis on the development of imaginative movies, pamphlets, and other materials for use in the public schools and in the mass media. Effective health education must begin in childhood. By the time an adult has developed a set of unwise habits, it is usually too late to influence him or her. Especially shocking—and in sharp contrast with the situation in countries like Denmark and New Zealand—is the evidence that many children and adults have no contact with dental care. Also shocking are the increasingly frequent reports of the use of drugs and alcohol by teen-agers in high school or

---

[8] See, especially, Fuchs (1974) and reports of research conducted under the direction of Dr. Lester Breslow at the School of Public Health, University of California, Los Angeles.

[9] See Section 7 for a discussion of this legislation.

even earlier. Overcoming these problems calls for a vigorous and sustained national effort.

Physicians, dentists, and other health professionals also need to place greater emphasis on educating patients to undertake more informed responsibility for their own care and treatment. The need for this type of emphasis is especially well exemplified in cases of hypertension, obesity, and diabetes. And, despite the pronounced improvement in scientific knowledge of the relationship between diet and heart problems, many adults do not become aware of these relationships until disaster strikes.

Urgent recommendation 5: *In the light of accumulating evidence that mortality rates in the United States are excessively high chiefly because of unwise personal habits and high accident rates, major emphasis should be placed in the coming years on the development of more effective programs of health education. Health professionals also need to be trained to place greater emphasis on educating patients to play a more active role in their own care and treatment.*

2

The 1971
Legislation

Its Provisions

The current controversies over health manpower legislation cannot be adequately interpreted without an acquaintance with the most important provisions of the landmark 1971 legislation.[1] These provisions included:

1. *Capitation grants for schools of medicine, osteopathy, and dentistry*
   a. $2,500 for each full-time first-, second-, and third-year student, plus $4,000 for each graduate from a four-year curriculum or $6,000 for each graduate from a three-year curriculum;
   b. $1,000 for each full-time student enrolled in a program for the training of physician's assistants or dental therapists;
   c. $1,000 for each enrollment bonus student (a member of a first-year class that exceeds certain enrollment standards. For example, the Fall 1971 first-year class must exceed the Fall 1970 first-year class by 5 percent or five students,

---

[1] Public Law 92-157, November 18, 1971. The legislation applied not only to schools of medicine, osteopathy, and dentistry, but also to certain other health-professions schools, such as schools of pharmacy, podiatry, and veterinary medicine. For reasons mentioned in the preface, we confine our discussion to schools of medicine, osteopathy, and dentistry.

whichever is greater. There are comparable provisions for subsequent years);
d. *But,* capitation payments are conditional on an increase in first-year enrollment of 10 percent over enrollment in the fall of 1970, if such enrollment was not more than 100, and of 5 percent or 10 students, whichever is greater, if such enrollment was more than 100.
e. *And* they are also conditional on a plan by the school to establish and carry out over the next two school years projects in at least three of such categories as improving or accelerating curriculum, developing interdisciplinary training, and the like.

2. *Grants for training, traineeships, and fellowships in family medicine*
Provides for grants to any public or nonprofit private hospital to develop and operate an approved training program in family medicine for medical students, interns, residents, or practicing physicians and to provide traineeships and fellowships for participants in such a program.

3. *Postgraduate training programs for physicians and dentists*
Provides for grants to schools of medicine, osteopathy, or dentistry and to public or nonprofit private hospitals to assist in meeting the educational costs of the first three years of graduate training programs in primary care or in any other area of health care that has a shortage of qualified physicians or dentists. Grants amount to $3,000 for each trainee, and applications must include evidence that the applicant has a program to encourage physicians and dentists to enroll in such programs and will increase the number of positions open in such programs.

4. *Special-project grants for health-professions schools*
Provides for grants for such purposes as curriculum improvements (with emphasis on programs for training in family medicine), interdisciplinary training, encouragement of enrollment of students likely to practice in shortage areas, encouragement of minority enrollment, preceptorships, and so on.

5. *Health-manpower education initiative awards*
Authorizes grants to public or private nonprofit health or

educational entities and contracts with public or private health or educational entities to (1) aid health-manpower shortage areas, (2) initiate or improve training of health personnel, (3) emphasize team approach to health delivery, (4) aid regional arrangements to carry out such purposes, and so on. It is under this provision that funds have been allocated to universities to develop area health education centers.

6. *Construction grants and start-up grants*
    a. Construction grants up to 80 percent of costs for new schools, major expansion of existing schools, and major remodeling or renovation projects; grants up to 70 percent of costs for other projects involving teaching facilities and, with certain qualifications, up to 50 percent for research facilities;
    b. Provisions for loan guarantees and interest subsidies;
    c. Start-up grants providing, in the year before a school enrolls students, $10,000 for each full-time student estimated to be enrolled in the following year, and gradually declining amounts in subsequent years.

7. *Student assistance*
    a. Scholarships. Annual maximum award per student, $3,500. Formula for appropriations provides, for fiscal 1972, an amount determined by multiplying $3,000 by 10 percent of enrollment, and, for fiscal 1973 and 1974, $3,000 multiplied by the number of disadvantaged students.
    b. Shortage-area scholarship programs. Special scholarships of up to $5,000 per year for students of medicine who agree to practice, after completion of professional training, in underserved areas, with priority of assistance to low-income students residing in underserved areas.
    c. Student loans. Annual maximum award per student, $3,500, with forgiveness provisions for students who, following completion of professional training, practice in underserved areas.
    d. Special traineeships and fellowships. For personnel in health-professions teaching, for training in family medicine, and for postgraduate medical and dental training.

Research funds, which represent a large proportion of federal aid to university health science centers, are provided under separate legislation, particularly in the form of funds for the National Institutes of Health.

Its Implementation

As in many areas of federal policy, the appropriations to implement the provisions of the 1971 legislation have fallen short of authorizations and of the intent of the law. Total federal funds received by medical schools increased steadily and substantially through 1973-74 and fell off slightly in the following year (Table A-1, Appendix). Federal funds for dental schools also rose through 1973-74, but fell off relatively more sharply in 1974-75 (Table A-2, Appendix). The more precipitate decline for dental schools partially reflects the fact that funds for research and graduate training are not included in the data provided by the American Association of Dental Schools (AADS), and thus the decline in capitation payments and other types of support had a more decisive impact on the total shown than in the case of medical schools, which received an increase in research funds in 1974-75.[2] Medical schools also received an increase in construction funds in that year, whereas dental schools experienced a decline.

Especially significant to an understanding of the impact of the 1971 legislation, however, is the large increase in capitation grants for both medical and dental schools between fiscal 1971 and fiscal 1972. Previously, capitation grants had been provided on a much smaller scale only to schools that were increasing their enrollment. Under the 1971 legislation, capitation grants were intended to flow to all schools, although they were made conditional on modest increases in enrollment. The appreciable decline in capitation grants in fiscal 1975 had a severe effect on the overall financial position of the schools.

This effect shows up clearly in terms of capitation payments per student. In current dollars, capitation payments per

---

[2]The increase was in current dollars; as indicated in Section 1, there was a decline in constant dollars.

M.D. candidate, for example, rose from $561 in fiscal 1970 to $1,972 in fiscal 1975 and then fell back to $1,537 in fiscal 1976. (The apparent inconsistency between this experience and the behavior of total funds for capitation in Table A-1 is explained by the forward-funding basis used for capitation payments—appropriations for a given fiscal year are used to provide payments for the following year.) The inadequacy of these amounts becomes especially apparent when we consider that full implementation of the provisions of the 1971 legislation would have provided payments well above $2,500 per student— the exact amount depending on the relationship between the number of three-year and four-year graduates and the number of enrollees in the first, second, and third years.

In view of the exacerbation of inflation in recent years, the impact of inadequate capitation payments on the medical schools can best be interpreted if the amounts are converted to constant dollars. In terms of 1967 dollars, the payments rose to a peak of about $1,475 in fiscal 1973 and fell back to about $930 in fiscal 1976.[3]

The 1971 legislation was intended to be effective for three years, and thus would have expired June 30, 1974, had it not been continued during the last several fiscal years, while Congress debated amendments. Under the legislative proposals now being considered (June 1976), capitation payments would be smaller than under the 1971 legislation and, as suggested in Section 1, would be subject to more stringent conditions. Before we proceed to a discussion of these proposals, we need to mention the desirability of continuing the present legislation through fiscal 1977—or for a year after the effective date of new legislation (whenever that will be). This has been suggested by numerous representatives of university health science centers, on the ground that the schools need assurance of a continued flow of federal funds, even though on the reduced basis of the last several years, while the procedures for implementing the new legislative provisions are developed by the Administration.

---

[3]We are indebted to the Association of American Medical Colleges for providing these data, as well as the data in Table A-1, Appendix.

Detailed recommendation 1: *The Council recommends extending the provisions of existing health-manpower legislation for a year after the effective date of revised legislation, in order to avoid a disruption of the flow of federal support funds to university health science centers.*

3

Shortages or Impending Surpluses?

In 1970, when the Carnegie Commission report on medical and dental education was published, there was widespread agreement that the United States suffered a shortage of physicians. Although the deficit of physicians was difficult to measure, four types of evidence indicated a shortage: (1) exceedingly high average incomes of physicians relative to those in most other professions, (2) long waiting lines for emergency services in hospital outpatient clinics, (3) the very long work week of the typical physician (with a median work week of 60 hours reported in 1968), and (4) the rising influx of foreign medical graduates (FMGs). There was also a serious geographic maldistribution of physicians and other health manpower, but this could not be interpreted as clear evidence of a general shortage, because it could have reflected a combination of surpluses in some areas and shortages in others.

Is There a Shortage of Physicians?

Even in 1970, however, a few medical economists argued that there was no general shortage of physicians, but only a problem of maldistribution and of overreliance on the skills of highly trained physicians, who could delegate some of their functions to physician's assistants and other allied health manpower. One problem with these arguments, however, was that it was unrealistic to suppose that established physicians would move from, say, New York to Mississippi to overcome geographic mal-distribution. Only through an increase in the supply of newly trained physicians and the development of financing and other policies that would induce them to practice in underserved areas could there be a realistic expectation of overcoming geographic maldistribution. And, although a few innovative training programs for physician's assistants were developed, the number of students involved in such programs in 1970 was very small.

The Increase in Aggregate Supply

Whether there exists a general shortage of physicians is now more widely disputed than it was in 1970. The increase in the size of medical-school entering classes has been more rapid than had been expected—from 11,300 in 1970 to 15,300 in 1975, or 35 percent. The rise exceeded the Carnegie Commission's most optimistic projection, which predicted an entering class of 14,700 in 1975 (Carnegie Commission, 1970, p. 42). The Commission recommended that the number of entrant places should be increased to 16,400 by 1978, and that demand and supply relationships should be reassessed then. It now appears probable that that figure will be reached, or possibly exceeded, by 1978.

Nearly all schools have increased the size of entering classes, with the largest percentage increases generally occurring in those schools with relatively small numbers of first-year students in the late 1960s (Table A-3, Appendix).

The rise in medical-school enrollment has also been accompanied by significant increases in the proportions of women and members of minority groups among medical-school entrants. For women, the rise was from 11 percent in 1970 to 24 percent in 1975. For disadvantaged minorities, the increase has been less spectacular and less steady—their proportion of entering students rose from 7 percent in 1970 to 10 percent in 1974 and then fell back to 9 percent in 1975 ("U.S. Medical School Enrollment . . . ," 1975, p. 304; and "Medical School Enrollment . . . ," 1976, p. 145).[1]

---

[1]Included among disadvantaged minorities are blacks, Native Americans, and Latinos. Not included are Chinese- and Japanese-Americans, whose

In projections prepared for the Carnegie Commission, Blumberg (1971) estimated (on the basis of the highest of three projections of the increase in medical-school entrants) that the ratio of active physicians to 100,000 population would rise from 147 in 1967 to 154 in 1972 and to 182 by 1987. The actual ratio in 1972 was 167.

More recently, in testimony before the Subcommittee on Health and the Environment, U.S. House of Representatives, the former secretary of HEW, Caspar W. Weinberger, indicated that the physician-population ratio would rise to between 207 and 217 in 1985 and commented that "these rates would place the United States near the top of all the industrialized nations in terms of overall physician supply" (Weinberger, 1975, p. 311). These estimates assumed a 40 percent reduction in the inflow of FMGs, because "increases in the numbers of U.S. graduates and the likely actions of both the private and public sectors in addressing the training of graduate physicians, both foreign and domestic educated, may well produce a downward trend in the influx of foreign medical graduates" (Weinberger, 1975, p. 312).[2]

Recently it has been shown that the increase in the number of FMGs entering the United States has been exaggerated through the practice of including those entering on temporary and permanent visas each year. As Stevens and others (1975) have shown, changes in immigration procedures have enabled an increasing number of FMGs who entered the country on temporary visas to change to immigrant (or permanent visa) status at a later point. These individuals, as a result, were double-counted when the annual data on those with temporary and with permanent visas were combined. Nevertheless, the adjusted statistics

---

proportion of medical-school students has tended to exceed their proportion of the total population for some years.

[2] The HEW estimate of the physician-population ratio for the mid-1980s exceeded Blumberg's for several reasons: (1) because population growth has continued to slow down since Blumberg's estimates were prepared and (2) because Blumberg assumed that the inflow of foreign medical graduates would cease after 1977 (an assumption based on the premise that the demand for FMGs would decline as the number of U.S. graduates increased). The ratios include active physicians and osteopaths.

developed by Stevens and her co-authors showed that the number of new entries of FMGs rose from 6,010 in 1965 to 8,120 in 1973, and that the number in the latter year was almost as large as in the peak year of 1968, when there were 8,400 new entries. But their adjusted data do not show the steady increase in the early 1970s that previously published data had shown, and their actual total of slightly more than 8,000 in 1973 is far below the 12,300 indicated by the unadjusted data for that year. Even so, the total continued to be sizable in comparison with the number of U.S. medical graduates, which amounted to 10,390 in 1973.

Another indication of the magnitude of the cumulative inflow of FMGs is the fact that they constitute about 30 percent of all house-staff physicians in U.S. hospitals (Figure 3) and about one-fifth of all U.S. physicians. This would be a matter of less concern if the FMGs came predominantly from countries in which standards of medical education were comparable to those in the United States, but a rising proportion has been coming from relatively underdeveloped countries, in some of which, at least, the standards of medical education are inferior to those in the U.S. Allegations that FMGs, on the average, perform much less well on comparable examinations than U.S. medical graduates have been disputed,[3] but there is no dispute over the great

---

[3]The report of a Task Force on Foreign Medical Graduates of the Association of American Medical Colleges stated that "in objective-type examinations FMGs perform at a lower level than do graduates from American medical schools" ("Graduates of Foreign Medical Schools . . . ," 1974, p. 816). This has been disputed by Stevens (1976, p. 77), who has argued that performance of FMGs and U.S. medical graduates on examinations cannot be compared, because the examinations taken by FMGs are rarely taken by U.S. medical graduates. However, the contention of Lee and others (1976) that the questions included in the Educational Council for Foreign Medical Graduates examination (discussed more fully in Section 4) could be correctly answered by the vast majority of U.S. medical students in their fourth year, seems reasonable. In contrast, only 40 percent of the FMGs taking the examination pass the first·time. In a statement at hearings on the maldistribution of physicians conducted by the U.S. Senate Subcommittee on Health in September 1975, Senator Edward M. Kennedy stated that only 20 percent of FMGs could pass the national board examinations passed by 89 percent of U.S. graduates (Kennedy, 1976, p. 925).

Figure 3. Internships and residencies in the United States, and positions
filled by United States and foreign graduates, 1949-50 to 1973-74

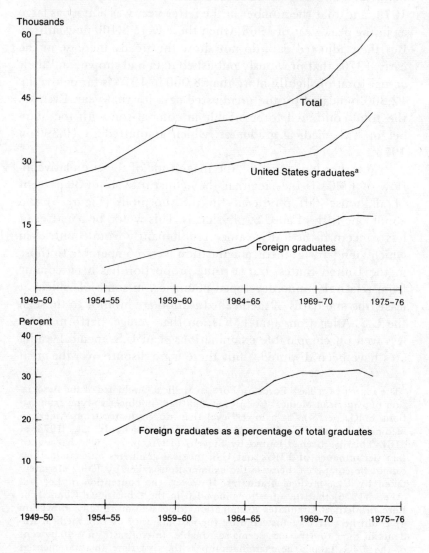

[a]Includes Canadian graduates.

Source: Computed from data in "Medical Education in the United States, 1973-74,"
(1975, p. 49).

variation in the performance of FMGs from different countries and from different schools within some countries.

Stevens and others (1975) showed that not only had previously published statistics overstated the number of FMGs entering the country, but that they had also overstated the increase in the proportion coming from Asia. Even so, of the adjusted total of nearly 6,700 entering the U.S. between 1965 and 1973, 48 percent came from Asia, while 23 percent came from Europe, 15 percent from North and Central America, 9 percent from South America, and 5 percent from other areas.

If the FMGs were employed primarily in underserved areas, the continued influx could be interpreted as helping to overcome geographic maldistribution. In 1970, however, FMGs represented the highest percentages of physicians in New York (35 percent), Rhode Island (30 percent), and Illinois (28 percent), which have tended to be states with comparatively high physician-population ratios, whereas FMGs tended to account for small proportions of physicians in most of the southern states, which have had the lowest physician-population ratios. Significantly, also, most of the FMGs are employed by hospitals or other institutions. Only about one-third of all FMGs were in office-based practice in 1970, compared with approximately two-thirds of the active physician graduates of U.S. and Canadian medical schools.[4] And particularly revealing as to the nature of the demand for FMGs is the fact that, in 1972, two-thirds of the FMG interns and residents were in programs not affiliated with a medical school. As Lee and others (1976) have pointed out, these unaffiliated hospitals are apparently more concerned with meeting staff requirements to maintain the daily operation of the facility than of providing a well-planned education program. Another important aspect of the employment of FMGs is that, in addition to the 68,000 included in the American Medical Association (AMA) registry in 1971, some

---

[4]Graduates of Canadian medical schools are usually grouped with graduates of U.S. medical schools and are not classified as FMGs. The data cited here on employment of FMGs are largely from Lee (1975) and Lee and others (1976).

10,000 to 19,000 unlicensed FMGs were employed in the United States, many of them in state institutions.

The heavy influx of FMGs would not have occurred in an absence of a demand for their services. The demand for medical care in the United States tended to increase throughout the postwar period, stimulated at first by the rapid spread of private health-insurance coverage and later by the enactment of Medicare and Medicaid legislation in 1965. These developments contributed to more adequate financing, among other things, of internships and residencies, because third-party reimbursement became available to cover their compensation wholly or partly. The enormous increase in the total number of internships and residencies is indicated clearly in Figure 3.

In 1965, Medicare and Medicaid brought about an accelerated demand for health care by providing public funds for services to the aged and the poor, many of whom had formerly lacked adequate services. There is considerable evidence that this accelerated increase in demand had its impact primarily in the years from 1965 to 1970, and that after that the increase in demand slowed down. Between 1973-74 and 1974-75, however, inflation in the costs of medical care was particularly pronounced, reflecting the general increase in inflationary pressure in the national economy (see the various series in Table 1).

What happens in the future will depend a good deal on whether national health-insurance legislation is enacted and whether that legislation is sufficiently comprehensive to bring about another sharp increase in the demand for medical care. At present, the conflict between advocates of sharply differing national health-insurance proposals does not seem likely to be resolved in the near future.

How reliable is the Administration's projection of a physician-population ratio of 207 to 217 per 100,000 population in 1985? It is based on a detailed projection prepared by the Bureau of Health Resources Development (BHRD—U.S. Public Health Service, 1974), indicating that the total number of active physicians (M.D.s and D.D.O.s) will rise to 494,100 (low projection) or 519,100 (basic methodology projection) by 1985. A high projection was also prepared but seems improbable for

Table 1. Selected measures relating to medical care, 1949-50 to 1974-75

Year	Health expenditures as percent of gross national product	Index of medical care costs (1967 = 100)	Consumer price index (1967 = 100)	Median net earnings of self-employed physicians	Ratio of physicians' earnings to median family incomes
1949-50	4.6%	53.2	71.8		
1954-55	4.6	64.1	80.4	$16,017 (1955)	3.62
1959-60	5.2	77.8	88.0	22,100 (1959)	4.08 (1959)
1964-65	5.9	88.4	93.7	28,670	4.24
1965-66	5.9	91.5	95.9	30,565	4.23
1966-67	6.2	98.6	98.6	33,450	4.32
1967-68	6.5	103.1	102.1	36,175	4.36
1968-69	6.7	109.8	107.0	39,085	4.33
1969-70	7.2	117.0	113.1	41,025	4.25
1970-71	7.6	124.5	118.8	42,100	4.18
1971-72	7.9	130.5	123.3	41,715	3.90
1972-73	7.8	135.1	129.2	41,435	3.58
1973-74	7.7	144.1	140.4		
1974-75	8.3	159.5	154.5		

Sources: U.S. Bureau of the Census (selected years); *Economic Report of the President, 1976*; U.S. Office of Management and Budget (1973); and Mueller and Gibson (1976).

a number of reasons. There are several problems with the low and basic projections:

1. The work was undertaken when the most recent firm figures on medical-school entrants and graduates were for 1970-71. Not surprisingly, both the low and basic projections understate the increase in the first half of the 1970s by a considerable margin and thus tend to understate the probable numbers of medical-school entrants and graduates in the latter half of the 1970s and the first half of the 1980s. The low

projection—particularly deficient in this respect—assumes that the number of entrants will reach 14,339 by 1974-75 and remain unchanged thereafter, while the number of graduates will reach 13,579 by 1977-78 and then stabilize.

2. On the other hand, the basic projection probably overstates the net increase in the number of FMGs practicing in the United States in future years, and assumes that the annual net increase will remain constant at 5,200 from 1971 to 1990. The low projection may be closer to the probable net increase, assuming an annual net inflow of 3,800 over the period. We believe, however, that as the number of U.S. graduates increases—and it is certain to increase rapidly in the next five to ten years—the demand for FMGs will decline and the net inflow will fall off gradually. It is certain to fall off if restrictions on the entry of FMGs are tightened.

Because of these deficiencies in the official projections—to a considerable extent attributable to the passage of time since the work on them was undertaken—we have developed our own projections. The results do not differ greatly from the BHRD projections, because the differences in assumptions have offsetting effects. In other words, we have projected a more pronounced growth in the number of medical-school entrants and graduates (Figure 4), but have assumed that the net annual inflow of FMGs will decline (at varying rates) and ultimately reach zero (in 1980 for the low projection and in 1987 for the high projection). FMGs would continue to enter on a visiting-scholar basis, but the number of temporary entrants would stabilize and result in no net addition to supply. Our methods are explained fully in Appendix B.

Whereas the BHRD projected that there would be 494,100 to 519,100 physicians by 1985, our projections indicate a supply of 491,000 to 510,000 by 1985. The U.S. Bureau of the Census has published revised population projections since the BHRD analysis was completed, and we present physician-population ratios based on Census Series II (Figure 2), arriving at ratios ranging from 210 to 218.[5] It is relevant to point out in

[5] We believe that Series II, which like the former Series E, assumes that the fertility rate will approach 2.1, is probably more realistic than Series I.

Figure 4. First-year enrollment in medical[a] and dental schools,
actual to 1975-76, projected to 1989-90 or 1986-87

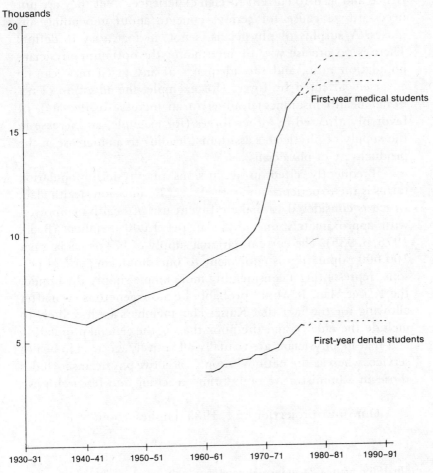

[a]Includes schools of osteopathy from 1960-61 on.

Sources: Fein (1967); "Medical Education in the United States, 1974-75," (1975, p. 1338); U.S. Public Health Service (1974); and Carnegie Council projections of medical school entrants.

this connection that the continued fall in the birthrate in the first half of the 1970s has slowed the rate of population growth substantially, and thus this factor alone would increase physician-population ratios based on earlier projections of physicians.

Physician-population ratios rising above 200 per 100,000 population are very high in relation to previous American experience and also to current foreign experience.[6] Yet they are not necessarily a cause for serious concern about impending surpluses. A surplus of physicians is not, in fact, easy to define. There is no precise way of determining the optimum physician-population ratio, and the adequacy of any given ratio can be adversely affected by forces (for example, the adoption of national health insurance) leading to an increase in demand, or favorably affected by other forces (for example, an increase in the supply of physician's assistants) leading to an increase in the productivity of physicians.

Frequently cited in discussions of physician-population ratios is the experience under the Kaiser Foundation Health Plan, which is considered to make efficient use of health manpower, with approximately one physician per 1,000 members (Beall, 1976, p. 935). The current national supply of 174 physicians per 100,000 population is equivalent to one physician per 574 persons, representing a considerably more ample supply than under the Kaiser Plan. It would probably be more generous even after allowing for the fact that Kaiser Plan members are less likely to include the elderly and the poor than is the general population and that its physicians are virtually all actively engaged in health service, whereas the national supply of active physicians includes those in administrative or full-time teaching and research positions.

Our low projection for 1985 implies about one active

---

[6] In 1969, among 24 industrial countries, only two had physician-population ratios exceeding 200 per 100,000 population—Israel, with 245, and the U.S.S.R., with 231 (Lee, 1975, p. 403). In both of these countries the situation is somewhat unusual, because of the large number of trained professionals among immigrants to Israel and because, with relatively fewer allied health professionals available, physicians in the Soviet Union perform functions that would not be considered suitable for physicians in the United States (Cooper, 1971, p. 417). The high ratio in the Soviet Union is not explained by the large numbers of *feldshers* (paramedical workers with no precise parallel in this country), who are not included in the statistics on physicians.

physician for every 477 persons.[7] Yet it is not clear that this implies a serious problem of surplus supply. A surplus of physicians would probably not manifest itself in unemployment among these highly trained professionals, but rather in some decline in their average incomes relative to the incomes of those in other professions and in a decline in their average hours of work, both of which have been exceedingly high.[8]

Increasing the likelihood of an overall surplus, however, is the currently rapid increase in the number of physician's assistants and nurse practitioners (discussed in the following section). Indeed, under conditions of rapidly increasing physician supply, rising emphasis on training physician extenders—however desir-

---

[7]Although we have characterized such a supply as unprecedented in the usually cited historical statistics, it was not unknown in colonial times. According to Stevens (1971, p. 14), the ratio of doctors to population in the Revolutionary era was 1 to 600, while an estimate for New York in 1750 gives a ratio of 1 to 350 and for Williamsburg in 1730 about 1 to 135. The standards of quality of training in colonial times, however, left much to be desired—with no medical schools, no licensing or other controls of quality, and apprenticeship as the usual method of training.

[8]The probability of a decline in relative incomes of physicians under conditions of rapidly increasing supply is disputed by some experts, citing evidence, such as that of Fuchs (1974, p. 73), that competition among surgeons in affluent suburbs that clearly have a surplus of surgeons does not drive surgeons' fees down. See, also, Feldstein (1970) for an analysis of the capacity of the physician to control both price and quantity of services under conditions of monopolistic competition and ethical restraints on price competition. It seems likely, however, that such perverse behavior of demand and supply is improbable except in relatively affluent communities. Health-insurance plans include ceilings on surgeons' fees, holding them to what is considered the prevailing rate, and only relatively affluent patients can afford to pay the difference between what the insurance plan allows and what the surgeon may actually charge. We have seen, also, that median net earnings of self-employed physicians leveled off after 1970, probably reflecting the rapid increase in the number of youthful physicians, and perhaps, also, the impact on net earnings of sharply increasing malpractice-insurance costs. Even so, the prevailing patterns of compensation under private health insurance and such government programs as Medicare and Medicaid encourage inflation in physicians' fees and even sharper inflation in hospital costs. For an excellent discussion of these influences, see Stevens (1971) and a recent article by Enthoven (1976), in which the author argues convincingly that effective control of costs in medical care will depend on expansion of prepaid health plans.

able it may be in terms of more effective use of health man-power—may be discouraged. Schools might find it difficult to raise the funds to support such programs in these circumstances.

An increase in the aggregate supply of physicians would probably ease shortages in underserved areas, although it is unlikely that an increase in supply alone, in the absence of other measures, would greatly alleviate this problem. The adequacy of any given physician-population ratio also cannot properly be interpreted without a consideration of what proportion of physicians are engaged in primary care. We shall discuss this more fully at a later point.

It has frequently been noted that projections may turn out to be wrong because they set in force reactions that tend to disprove their validity. This could happen in the case of the supply of physicians if, for example, the net inflow of FMGs fell off more abruptly and more drastically than we have assumed. However, increasingly the rise in the number of U.S. medical graduates will become the predominant force in the supply of physicians. Even if the net inflow of FMGs were to be zero from 1976 on, our low projection of U.S. medical graduates would imply 477,000 physicians by 1985, compared with about 350,000 in 1973.

The fear of an impending surplus could also discourage increasing numbers of young people from seeking a career in medicine. Undoubtedly there will be some tendency in this direction as the supply of physicians increases, but there will be some powerful counterforces as well:

1. The number of applicants to medical schools has increased much more rapidly than the number of admissions. The ratio of applicants to admitted first-year students rose from about 2.0 in the late 1960s to 2.8 in 1974-75, and substantial numbers of disappointed applicants have been seeking medical education abroad ("Medical Education in the United States, 1974-75," 1975, pp. 1336-1343). Thus, the number of applicants could continue to be quite large in relation to available

student places, even if the ratio of applicants to admitted students fell back considerably.[9]

2. Even with a substantial increase in the aggregate supply of U.S.-trained physicians, problems of geographic maldistribution and shortages of primary-care physicians are likely to remain serious enough, as we have suggested, to call for continued efforts to train substantial numbers of young physicians.

3. Adoption of a comprehensive national health-insurance system could lead to another decisive increase in the demand for health care and in the aggregate demand for physicians' services. It is sometimes argued that the great majority of Americans are already covered by private health insurance or by federal programs, such as Medicare and Medicaid, but, in fact, nearly 40 percent of the population under age 65 did not have coverage for physicians' office and home visits in 1964, while 20 percent did not have coverage for hospital care (Mueller and Piro, 1976, p. 4). Outside of New York and California, moreover, Medicaid programs, which depend on the provision of matching funds by the states, tend to be very restrictive. In 1974, New York and California accounted for 36 percent of all medical assistance expenditures (U.S. Bureau of the Census, 1975, p. 308), compared with 19 percent of the population.[10]

As long as there is an appreciable inflow of FMGs, we can-

---

[9] Beginning in the early 1980s, the size of the 22-year-old population, from which medical-school applicants tend to be drawn, will begin to decline, and this could well mean a decline in absolute numbers of medical-school applicants even if the proportion of the 22-year-old population applying did not change. Past fluctuations in the number of medical-school applicants have been closely related to changes in the size of the 22-year-old population ("Medical School Admissions . . . ," 1975).

[10] Lee and others (1976) cite several studies that have attempted to estimate the impact of various national health-insurance proposals on the demand for physicians' and hospital services and conclude that most national health-insurance programs would have a significant impact on the requirements for physicians.

not be indifferent to the need to ensure that the increase in the number of U.S. graduates does not suffer a reversal. And we would reiterate the Carnegie Commission's statement (1970, p. 36) that "looking toward the future, the United States should become a net exporter of medical manpower, as part of the effort to raise the quality of medical education and medical care in underdeveloped countries."

Before leaving the question of aggregate supply, we need to consider briefly the views of those who have argued for some years that an increase in the supply of physicians is not needed and would contribute little or nothing to improving the health of Americans. Probably the most effective spokesperson for this point of view has been Victor Fuchs, especially in a recent volume in which he stated (1974, p. 16):

> The chief killers today are heart disease, cancer, and violent deaths from accidents, suicide, and homicide. The behavioral component in all these causes is very large, and until now medical care has not been very successful in altering behavior.

This is an extremely important point, and it has been stressed by other experts who have analyzed the problem of lower life-expectancy in the United States, especially among males, than in a number of other advanced countries. It underlies the emphasis we have given in Section 1 to health education. Yet the victims of the "killer" diseases do benefit from prompt and competent medical care. Moreover, Fuchs has nothing to say about the financial problems of medical schools or how to maintain the quality of medical education and research in the face of those problems.

Far more extreme are the views of Illich (1976), who argues that modern medical care often does more harm than good for patients. While Illich's views are provocative and call attention to many serious defects in health care, the reader has a distinct impression, at times, that he would take us back to the nineteenth century and erase all the progress in medical knowledge that has been made in the present century. Moreover, he tends to blame the medical profession for problems that are by no means wholly the fault of physicians. Overhospitalization, for example, is related to the type of health-insurance plan to which patients belong. Several studies have shown lower hospital use by subscribers to prepaid group-practice plans (Klarman, 1965, p. 130).

Geographic Disparities

There has long been a serious problem of geographic differences in the supply of physicians and other health manpower. The supply has tended to be largest in relation to population in the New England, Middle Atlantic, and Pacific states. It has been least favorable in the East South Central and West South Central states (Figure 5). Generally, the differences have been related to differences in per capita income and in degree of urbanization among the regions. Between 1965 and 1974, the ratio of physicians to population increased in all of the regions, but the pattern of variations remained little changed.

Disparities among individual states are even more pronounced than among regions, ranging from 84 physicians per 100,000 population in South Dakota to 249 in New York in 1974. Mississippi and some of the other southern states have historically ranked at or near the bottom of the scale and continue to do so. Even more critical are the deficiencies of supply in rural areas, which have been growing more serious. Between 1968 and 1973, smaller nonmetropolitan counties experienced actual numerical losses of physicians and declines in their physician-population ratios (Nesbitt and Ruhe, 1975, p. 522).

Less easy to document statistically, but generally accepted as a serious problem, is the deficiency of supply of physicians in the ghetto areas of large cities, where residents tend to depend on crowded hospital outpatient clinics, rather than on private physicians, for medical care.[11]

As has frequently been pointed out, however, differences

---

[11]A study by Dewey (1973) indicated that the inner suburban areas of Chicago had 123 physicians per 100,000 population in 1973, compared with only 75 for the inner-city area, not including the Loop. The ratio in the inner-city area had been 111 per 100,000 in 1950. Change in the socioeconomic status of the patient population was found to be the single most important factor in relocation of physicians.

Figure 5. Active physicians and dentists[a] per 100,000 population, by region, 1965 and 1973 or 1974

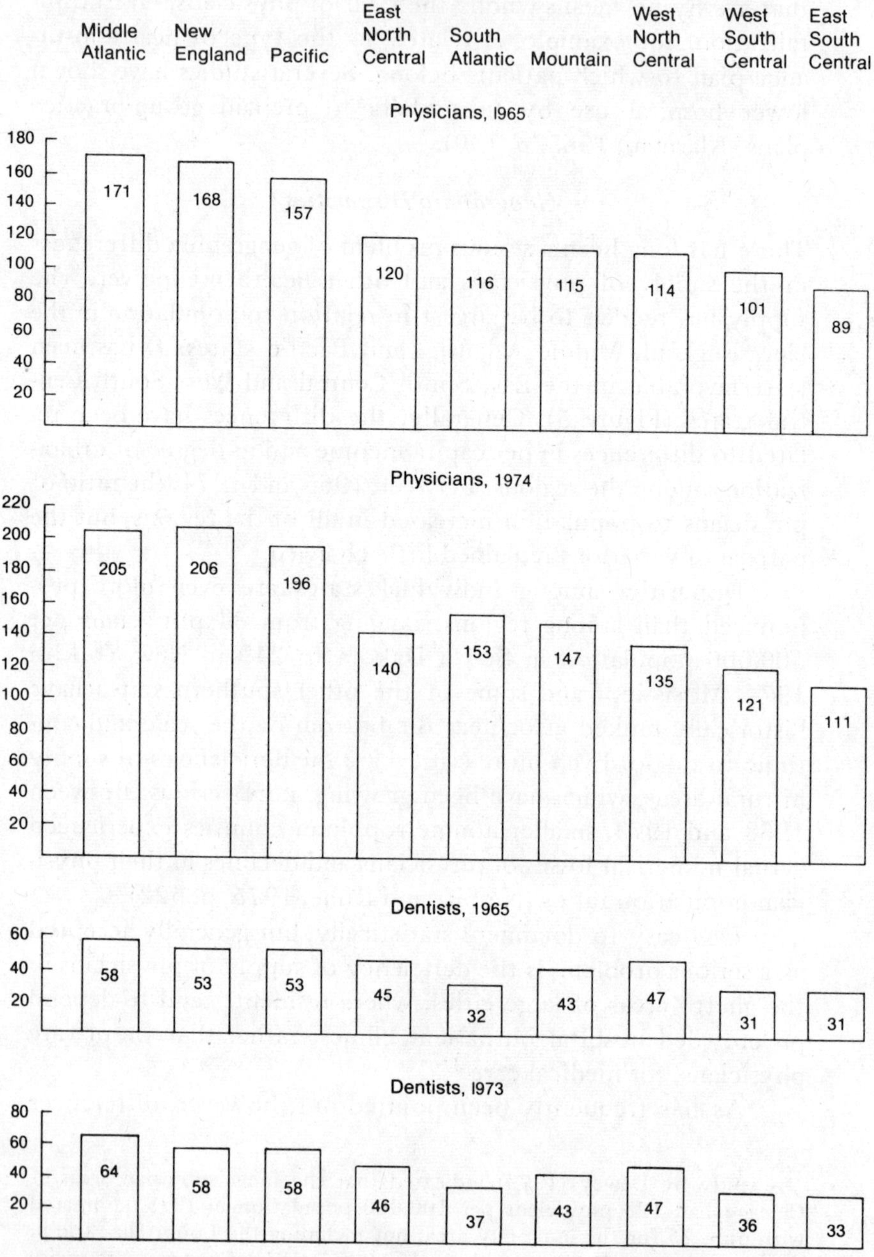

	Middle Atlantic	New England	Pacific	East North Central	South Atlantic	Mountain	West North Central	West South Central	East South Central
Physicians, 1965	171	168	157	120	116	115	114	101	89
Physicians, 1974	205	206	196	140	153	147	135	121	111
Dentists, 1965	58	53	53	45	32	43	47	31	31
Dentists, 1973	64	58	58	46	37	43	47	36	33

[a]Data do not include physicians and dentists in federal service; they also do not include doctors of osteopathy.

Sources: Computed from data in U.S. National Center of Health Statistics (annual); and American Medical Association (1975).

in physician-population ratios provide only a crude measure of differences in access to services. Some rural areas, especially in the South, are characterized by very low per capita incomes, whereas this is not nearly so true in the rural areas of the Middle West, and low income may be a more serious obstacle to access to medical care than distance. A resident of a rural area can frequently travel 50 miles in less time than it would take for a resident of a crowded urban area to travel 10 miles. A recent study by Held and Reinhardt (1975) indicated that disparities in access to care among areas with significant differences in their physician-population ratios were less pronounced than mere comparison of these ratios would suggest. Physicians in the shortage areas included in their study made up to 30 percent more patient visits per week and used 10 to 30 percent more auxiliary personnel than physicians in areas with relatively high physician-population ratios.[12]

As we shall see in later sections, some of the programs aimed at helping to overcome geographic disparities, such as the National Health Service Corps and the development of area health education centers, have been oriented more toward rural shortages than toward inner-city shortages. There needs to be more stress on the problems of underserved inner-city areas.

We believe, as indicated in Section 1, that geographic maldistribution of health manpower will be overcome only with great difficulty and through a combination of policies that will tend to induce, but not compel, physicians and other health professionals to locate in underserved areas.

We shall have more to say about federal implementation of these policies in subsequent sections.

The Supply of Primary-Care Physicians

The growth of specialization and the gradual decline in the supply of general practitioners have been predominant trends in American medicine in the twentieth century. They have been encouraged by the relatively high earning capacity and prestige

---

[12]For a more extensive discussion of these relationships, see Lee and others (1976).

of specialists, by the proliferation of specialties as medical knowledge has advanced, by the emphasis on the treatment of specialized cases in university teaching hospitals, and indeed, by the general atmosphere of the "Flexner model" medical school. They have also been encouraged by the tendency for private health-insurance plans to provide for hospital care and medical services in the hospital much more frequently than for physician's office or home visits, although these patterns have slowly been changing. Reimbursement policies under the federal Medicare and Medicaid programs have likewise been a factor.

Between 1931 and 1963, the number of general practitioners fell from 112,000 to 73,000, or from 72 to 28 percent of all physicians (Fein, 1967, pp. 68-72; and Table A-4, Appendix). In recent years, however, the new specialty of family practice, requiring three years of residency training, has developed. In addition, it has become customary to classify internists, pediatricians, and frequently, also, obstetricians and gynecologists, as primary-care physicians—a custom that recognizes the fact that these specialists have replaced the general practitioner, especially in urban areas, in the primary treatment of most patients. Thus, in analyzing recent trends, it is useful to distinguish between those physicians who are predominantly engaged in primary care and those specialists who usually treat patients on a referral basis.

Using this classification, we find that, as the total number of physicians increased sharply between 1963 and 1970, the proportion engaged in primary practice declined from about 55 to 44 percent, while the proportion in specialized practices increased (Table A-4, Appendix).[13] There have also been several studies that have indicated surpluses of surgeons (chiefly in affluent areas) and the probability of excessive numbers of surgical operations (Bunker, 1970; and Lewis, 1969). The decline

[13]These percentages must be interpreted with caution, because some of those in internal medicine, pediatrics, and obstetrics/gynecology are subspecialists and are not engaged in primary care. However, it has been estimated that 75 percent of all internists, for example, spend more than one-half of their time in primary care and 85 percent spend at least some time in primary care (Lee and others, 1976).

in the proportion engaged in primary practice was reversed between 1970 and 1973, however, primarily because of an increase in the percentage engaged in internal medicine.

A more sensitive measure of recent and current changes is the distribution of first-year residencies by field of specialization, for the distribution of all practicing physicians can change only slowly, and any change results chiefly from changes in the choices of beginning physicians. During the 1960s these choices tended to enhance the trend toward specialization (Table A-5, Appendix). In recent years, there has been a substantial change, but the data must be interpreted with caution, as the American Medical Association (AMA) discontinued publication of separate data on interns in 1974, because internships were to be integrated with first-year residencies by the end of the 1974-75 academic year.[14] Thus, beginning in 1974, data on internships were combined with data on first-year residencies, but data for earlier years were not revised to make them comparable. The proportion of first-year residents choosing primary-care types of residencies rose from 37.5 percent in 1970 to 43.8 percent in 1973. According to Lee and others (1976), adding internships that emphasized primary care raised the proportion to 56 percent of all first-year positions in the latter year. According to later AMA data, 55 percent of U.S. graduates in first-year residencies in 1974 and 58 percent in 1975 were in primary-care residencies (Nesbitt, Ruhe, and Peterson, 1976, p. 2039). Considerably more impressive are the recent data from the National Internship and Residency Matching Program, which indicate that, in the fall of 1976, 69 percent of U.S. graduates in first-year residencies will be in primary-care residencies (data provided by the AAMC).

Although it is important not to exaggerate the extent of the change and to recognize that some first-year residents shift

[14]This reflected the implementation of the AMA decision in 1970 to abolish "free standing" internships that were not integrated with residency programs. The change was made largely in recognition of the fact that increasing proportions of interns had been selecting specialties and spending at least part of the internship year in specialty training ("Medical Education in the United States, 1970-71," 1971).

their specialties in later years, a substantial change does appear to be under way. It has occurred in the absence of federal controls over residencies, along the lines of proposals currently before Congress (to be discussed in the following section). A number of influences have been at work to produce this change —the grants of $3,000 per postgraduate trainee in primary care under the 1971 legislation, special federal grants to support the establishment of family-practice residencies, state support for family-practice residency programs in public medical schools (see Section 8), and the tendency for many of the new medical schools established since 1967 to emphasize residencies in primary care. In addition, the increased emphasis on developing residency training in area health education centers and other geographically disbursed clinical-training centers has been a significant factor, for much of this training is in primary care. These developments will be discussed fully in Section 7.

Is There a Shortage of Dentists?

The available evidence suggests that the gap between the effective demand for dental care and the need that would exist if the entire population received adequate dental care has been wider than in the case of physicians. This is because a very substantial proportion of the population does not receive the regular dental care that is necessary for proper maintenance of healthy teeth. As recently as early 1975, at the annual meeting of the American Association of Dental Schools, a dental educator stated that "the majority of Americans who live out their normal life spans will lose all of their natural teeth" (Watkins, 1975, p. 10).[15] The most recent national survey of health, indicated that in 1974 about 10 percent of the population had never visited a dentist and another 14 percent had not visited a dentist for five years or more (U.S. Department of Health, Education, and Welfare, 1975a, p. 24). The average number of annual dental visits per person was 1.7, as contrasted with 4.9 physician visits per per-

---

[15] A 1967 report indicated that the percentage of the population with no natural teeth rose sharply with advancing age to 56 and 66 percent, respectively, for men and women aged 75 to 79 (U.S. Department of Health, Education and Welfare, 1967).

son (U.S. Department of Health, Education, and Welfare, 1975a, pp. 23, 25), and a large proportion of these visits is concentrated within a small percentage of the population. In view of the fact that dentists who encourage regular care for their patients typically arrange for three visits a year for each patient, the average number of visits per dentist would clearly have to rise considerably before an adequate standard of dental care could be reached.[16]

In 1970, there was considerably less evidence of a shortage of dentists (in relation to effective demand) than of a shortage of physicians. Dentists' hours of work, for example, tended to be much shorter than those of physicians, and almost no foreign dental school graduates were employed in United States dentistry. The movement toward private insurance for dental care was still in its infancy, however, compared with insurance for medical care. Only 6 percent of the population had private insurance coverage for dental care, compared with 76 percent for hospital care, 74 percent for surgical services, and 33 percent for office and home visits of physicians. Coverage of dental care under employee-benefit plans has spread quite rapidly since 1970, and by 1974, 16 percent of the population had some insurance coverage for dental care (Mueller and Piro, 1976, p. 4). To what extent the spread of such coverage, which can be dated from about 1965, is responsible is not clear, but the rise in net earnings of self-employed dentists from 1965 to 1975 was spectacular. Whereas, in 1965, median net earnings of self-employed dentists were $12,650, or only 44 percent of median net earnings of physicians, by 1972, median net dentists' earnings were $32,500 or about 80 percent of the corresponding figure for physicians (U.S. Bureau of the Census, 1975, p. 77).

There is little question that private health-insurance coverage for dental care will continue to spread, and a number of

---

[16]Patients who receive regular dental care frequently see a dental hygienist rather than the dentist, so that the three visits need not involve the dentist in all cases. In fact, in national statistics on dental visits, a visit is "any visit to a dentist's office for treatment including services by a technician or hygienist acting under a dentist's supervision." The definition of a physician's visit is similar, but may also include a telephone consultation.

national health-insurance proposals call for gradual coverage of dental care, usually beginning with coverage of children. Thus, the per capita demand for dental services is likely to rise. However, a continued rise in productivity of the average dentist is likely to be a moderating force. The use of dental assistants is quite common, and employment of dental hygienists and dental laboratory technologists has been growing rapidly. In 1970, there were 157,800 of these allied dental personnel, compared with 102,220 dentists.

The rise in the number of first-year dental students has not been as pronounced as that of medical students, but it has been substantial—from 4,560 in 1970-71 to 5,763 in 1975-76, or 26 percent (U.S. Public Health Service, 1974, p. 83; and American Dental Association, 1975, p. 9). Whereas women represented only about 1 percent of all dental students in the late 1960s, they accounted for 12 percent of first-year dental students in 1975-76. Disadvantaged minorities, who had also accounted for a very small percentage of dental students in the 1960s, made up 8 percent of entering students in 1975-76.[17]

The number of dental schools has been increasing slowly. In 1975-76, there were 59 schools with students enrolled, compared with 53 in 1970. We shall consider the location of dental schools in Section 6.

Projecting the future supply of dentists is somewhat less complicated than predicting the supply of physicians, because of the absence of any inflow of foreign dental graduates. In 1970, only 0.7 percent of active dentists were graduates of foreign dental schools, and most of these were graduates of Canadian schools (U.S. Public Health Service, 1974, p. 79). Even so, the behavior of future demand for dental care is uncertain, as are the relative roles of fully trained dentists and dental assistants of one kind or another in providing that care.

The BHRD projection of dentists is quite conservative, assuming that first-year dental-school enrollment will rise to

[17]We include here blacks, Latinos, Native Americans, and "other" minorities. Not included are Asians, who accounted for 3.2 percent of the 1975-76 entering class (American Dental Association, 1975, p. 4).

5,850 in 1978-79 and then level off. The most recent firm data on first-year enrollment at the time the projection was developed were for 1971-72, and there have been pronounced increases since then. As we have seen, first-year enrollment in 1975-76 was 5,763, whereas the BHRD projection for that year was 5,540. Underlying the BHRD assumption that first-year enrollment would level off after 1978-79 was an assumption that, when the 1971 health-manpower legislation expired in 1974, "there would be no extension of Federal legislative inducements to increase enrollments and the level of support from the public and private sectors combined would be sufficient only to maintain enrollment levels resulting from earlier Federal legislation" (U.S. Public Health Service, 1974, p. 82).

Despite its conservative assumptions, the projection does indicate an increase in the dentist-population ratio from an estimated 52.1 per 100,000 in 1975 to 58.9 in 1985 and 61.8 in 1990 (Figure 2). The 1985 ratio would be somewhat larger, as we saw in the case of physicians, on the basis of the Census Bureau's most recent Series II population projection.

Although we have not attempted a revision of the BHRD projection of dentists, there are reasons for believing that it may understate the increase in the supply of dentists. Annual reports on dental education do not provide data on ratios of applicants to admissions as do the annual reports on medical education, but it seems likely that the ratio has been rising. Thus there is likely to be pressure on dental schools to admit more students.

The continued spread of dental insurance—a virtual certainty—will increase the demand for dental services, but increased use of allied dental workers could hold down the rise in demand for fully trained dentists. In an attempt to assess various influences on the future demand for dentists, Wechsler, Williams, and Thum (1972a) conducted a survey of dental school deans and found that approximately three-fourths of the deans thought that by 1980 the number of dentists using auxiliary personnel "at chairside" would greatly increase, as would dental-insurance coverage. On the other hand, nearly one-half of the deans thought that fluoridation of more water supplies would hold down the demand for dental care, while 36 percent thought that a greater proportion of dentists in group practice would be a factor increasing dental productivity.

Geographic Maldistribution and Specialization

As Figure 5 shows, the pattern of regional differences in the ratio of dentists to population is very similar to that for physicians, and, in fact, a similar pattern prevails for all types of health manpower. We believe that the policies needed for alleviating these differences are much the same for dentists as for physicians. For example, emphasis on providing part of the training of dentists in area health centers could contribute to more effective geographic distribution of future practicing dentists.[18]

The growth of specialization in dentistry has not, until recently, been a matter of serious concern, as it has in medicine. Limited as dental responsibility is to the region of the mouth, the scope for proliferation of specialties is relatively narrow. Even so, the proportion of specialists among dentists rose from 3.6 percent in 1955 to 10.4 percent in 1973 (U.S. Public Health Service, 1974, pp. 79 and 82; and U.S. Senate, 1976, p. 57). As the demand for dental care rises, this proportion will also probably continue to increase. In fact, the marked trend toward specialty training among recent dental-school graduates (Shira, 1976, p. 2067) is becoming a matter of growing concern in dental education.

---

[18]In an analysis of maldistribution of dental manpower, Wechsler, Williams, and Thum (1972b) referred to the Carnegie Commission's proposal for area health education centers as one of the steps needed to attract dentists to underserved areas and also recommended active recruitment of dental students, along with provision of financial assistance for such students, from low-income areas.

4

Federal Capitation
Payments and
Related Policies

If federal support of medical and dental education is to provide the stable floor of financing that we consider essential, it should represent a stable proportion of the costs of education per student, with the remaining costs to be met by other public and private sources, including tuition. Thus the dollar amount would rise on the basis of a careful analysis indicating that costs of education had actually increased—not on the basis of a more general measure, such as the consumer price index, which might or might not be related to actual costs of health professions education. It should be kept in mind, in this connection, that medical schools receive income from patient care and from research activities. The income from patient care might well be increased under a national health-insurance program, as it has been under Medicare, Medicaid, and the spread of private health-insurance coverage. Thus, although gross educational costs will undoubtedly continue to increase, net educational costs will not necessarily increase proportionately.

We now have more adequate information on costs of education in the health professions than was available at the time the 1971 legislation was enacted. That legislation mandated a study of costs, which was carried out by the Institute of Medicine of the National Academy of Sciences. The resulting report (National Academy of Sciences, 1974) estimated average annual gross education costs per medical student at $12,650 in 1972-73, although costs among schools (calculated in an intensive analysis of a sample of schools) varied from $6,900 to $18,650.[1] These costs included the three components generally recognized as contributing to medical education: the teaching component, the patient-care component, and the research component. They did not include the costs of all patient care or research activities of a medical school, of course, but only those that contributed to the M.D. candidate's education. Deducting the income received from research and patient-care components, the Institute of Medicine arrived at average net costs of $9,700, with a range of $5,150 to $14,150 in 1972-73. Net costs of other health-professions schools were lower, ranging from $3,050 for schools of pharmacy to $7,400 for dental schools. The estimate of average net costs for schools of osteopathy was lower than for medical schools or dental schools, at $7,000.[2]

Basic Principles

We believe that capitation payments amounting to one-third of estimates of net educational costs per full-time student, as revised from time to time by an agency like the Institute of Medicine, would represent an appropriate contribution by the federal government to the costs of health-professions education, with the remaining costs to be contributed by state government and private sources, including student tuition. We do not believe however, that these payments should be entirely unconditional.

[1] The Carnegie Commission (1970, p. 69) estimated, on the basis of data available at the time, that annual educational costs per student ranged from $6,000 to $15,000 or $16,000. A study completed by the Association of American Medical Colleges in 1973 estimated that costs ranged from $16,000 to $26,000 in 1972 dollars (Association of American Medical Colleges, 1973, p. 1).

[2] The study also included schools of nursing, where net costs were estimated to average $1,500 for diploma schools, $1,650 for schools granting associate degrees, and $2,450 for baccalaureate programs.

We suggest that approximately one-sixth of net educational costs per student should be available to the schools on minimal conditions—maintenance of enrollment and expenditures from nonfederal sources should be the only important conditions. These payments would be regarded as the federal government's basic unconditional subsidy in recognition of the social benefits flowing from maintenance of high-quality medical and dental education.[3] Additional payments, amounting to one-sixth of educational costs per student, would be provided in the form of bonuses designed to achieve specific objectives.

Detailed recommendation 2: *To implement Urgent Recommendation 1, basic capitation payments amounting to one-sixth of net educational costs per full-time M.D. and D.D.S. candidate, as determined by an appropriate official body, should be provided each year to medical and dental schools. These payments should be subject only to reasonable conditions requiring maintenance of enrollment and of expenditures from nonfederal sources.*

Before specifying the purposes for which bonuses would be provided, we need to consider certain controversial proposals that have been under congressional consideration in the last few years—proposals that we believe would involve the federal government in an undesirable degree of detailed control over medical and dental education policies.

---

[3] The Institute of Medicine's report (National Academy of Sciences, 1974) proposed that one-third of net educational costs would be an appropriate standard for federal capitation payments. Later, both Lee (1975, p. 427) and the Association of American Medical Colleges (AAMC—Cooper, J. A. D., 1975, p. 469) proposed that the one-third would be a maximum attainable only by schools undertaking additional activities directed toward increasing the aggregate supply of physicians or physician extenders, as well as toward overcoming problems of geographic maldistribution and overemphasis on training for certain specialties. Schools not undertaking such projects would receive only 20 percent of net costs under the Lee proposal and one-half of the maximum amount (that is, 16.7 percent of net costs) under the AAMC proposal.

Capitation Payback Proposals

Especially controversial among recent legislative proposals have been those calling for repayment by medical and dental students of capitation payments made to their schools on behalf of their education. The bill (H.R. 5546) that was passed by the House of Representatives in July 1975, for example, would make capitation payments to schools of medicine, osteopathy, and dentistry conditional on assurances by the school that it would "enter into a legally enforceable agreement with each student enrolled in the school" after June 30, 1976 "under which the student agrees to pay, in equal annual installments . . . to the United States an amount equal to the total amount which the school received . . . because of the enrollment of the student in the school . . . ." The number of annual installments is to equal the number of fiscal years in which the school received a grant on account of the enrollment of the student, but payment need not begin until after completion of internship and residency, and will be excused for each year of service in the National Health Service Corps or in professional practice in an area that the Secretary of HEW has designated as a medically underserved area.

This provision was also included in a bill approved by the Senate Committee on Labor and Public Welfare in 1974, but was rejected on the floor of the Senate. It was not included in the bill approved by the Senate Committee on Labor and Public Welfare in April 1976, which called, instead, for each school to reserve a certain proportion of its student places for students who held National Health Service Scholarships committing them to serve for a period following graduation in underserved areas.

We do not favor capitation payback provisions as an approach to the problem of geographic maldistribution of physicians and dentists, for the following reasons:

1. Basic capitation payments should be regarded as a contribution to be made on a continuous basis by the federal government in recognition of the social benefits flowing from maintaining and improving the quality of medical and dental schools. They should not be regarded as payments on behalf

of individual students, giving rise to an obligation for repayment by those students.

2. The school's assurances of commitments on the part of students to practice in underserved areas would be exceedingly difficult for the schools to enforce following graduation of their students, and would impose a compulsory obligation on health-professions students not paralleled by similar obligations on students training for other occupations.

3. The acceptance by a student of special types of student aid that must be repaid if the student does not practice in an underserved area following graduation represents a preferable way of attempting to encourage more graduates of health-professions schools to practice in those areas, because it calls for a voluntary act on the part of the student and is associated with aid received by him or her, and not with payments made to his or her school.

4. The problem of overcoming geographic maldistribution calls for a combination of policies, as suggested in Section 3.

Enrolling National Health Service Corps Scholarship Holders

Opposition to the capitation payback proposals has led to proposals to require health-science schools to reserve a certain proportion of their student places for holders of National Health Service Corps (NHSC) scholarships as a condition for receiving capitation payments. These scholarships, which carry an obligation for a certain period of service in the corps, have become by far the most significant type of aid for medical and dental students in the major bills considered in the last several years. Under the bill approved by the Senate Labor and Public Welfare Committee in April 1976, schools of medicine and osteopathy must provide assurance that the following proportions of full-time students (excluding fourth-year students) have submitted applications and have agreed to accept NHSC scholarships—25 percent in 1977-78, 30 percent in 1978-79, and 35 percent in 1979-80.[4] For dental schools, the provisions call for reserving

---

[4]This type of requirement was first proposed by the Ford Administration in September 1975 (Cooper, 1976) and was included in legislation introduced for the Administration by Senator Kennedy in December

20 percent of first-year student places for NHSC scholarship holders in each of the three years (U.S. Senate, 1976, p. 184).

Capitation payments subject to these and other conditions would amount to $1,800 per student in 1978-79, $1,900 in 1979-80, and $2,000 in 1980-81. These payments would be approximately one-sixth of net educational costs per student in medical schools, in contrast with provisions for payments equalling approximately one-third of net costs in earlier Senate proposals.[5] The other conditions for capitation payments imposed by the bill will be discussed at a later point.

Although the policy of requiring a school to reserve a certain proportion of its student places for holders of NHSC scholarships is less objectionable than capitation payback provisions, it is contrary to the principle we have emphasized: that is, that basic capitation payments should be made in recognition of the social benefits of medical and dental education and should be subject only to minimal conditions. In addition, there is no assurance that NHSC scholarship holders will be evenly distributed among applicants to particular schools, among geographic regions, or among students of various ability levels. To some degree, the bill guards against these problems by providing that, if the assured national goal for each academic year is met, the provisions will not be enforced against individual schools, but this safeguard is dependent on a sufficient flow of applications for the NHSC scholarships.

We believe that a preferable approach is to provide a bonus amounting to one-sixth of net educational costs to a school for

---

1975. As reported by the Senate Subcommittee on Health, the requirements in the bill concern first-year students. However, the AAMC favored having the requirements apply to the student body as a whole, on the ground that this would involve less interference with the schools' admissions policies (Bennett and Cooper, 1976, p. 2055). At that time the percentages under discussion were 15, 20, and 25. The legislation was amended by the full Senate Committee on Labor and Public Welfare to apply to all students except those in the fourth year (Association of American Medical Colleges, 1976b).

[5] Annual net costs of education per student may be presumed to have risen from $9,700, as estimated by the Institute of Medicine in 1972-73, to about $10,800.

each NHSC scholarship holder admitted. This would provide a strong incentive to a school to attract such applicants, without imposing mandatory requirements. This approach would also be consistent with the general principle we have emphasized, under which each school would receive its basic one-sixth with minimal conditions and an additional one-sixth as a bonus tied to certain objectives.

Thus far, as we shall see in Section 5, there have been far more applicants for NHSC scholarships than the number of awards available. Whether this trend will continue when the number of scholarships is greatly increased, as contemplated under current legislative proposals, is not certain, but the scholarships are generous, and there is no evidence as yet that applications will not rise as scholarship funds increase. If this were to fail to happen, more stringent provisions could be considered, but there is a strong case at present for giving the incentive approach an adequate trial before considering mandatory requirements.

Enrollment Expansion?

The 1971 legislation, as we saw in Section 2, required increases in first-year enrollment as a condition of capitation payments. The sharp increase in the size of first-year medical-school classes in the first half of the 1970s tends to remove the need for such provisions, except to bring very small schools up to a more economical size, and for that purpose we suggest bonuses to induce expansion, rather than a provision making capitation payments conditional on expansion. In other words, we suggest a provision under which a medical school with an entering class under 100 would receive a bonus amounting to one-sixth of net educational costs for each student admitted over the number admitted in the preceding year until an entering class size of 100 is achieved. An increase of at least 10 percent in any given year, however, would be required before any bonuses could be paid. There remains the serious question, which we shall consider in Section 6, of whether such bonuses should be provided for all of the new medical schools that have reached an advanced planning stage but have not yet enrolled any students.

The situation of dental schools is somewhat different. Their expansion has been less pronounced, and the likelihood of a continued pronounced increase in the demand for dental services, in *relation* to the probable increase in the supply of dentists, is quite high.[6] Some dental educators, however, believe the primary need is for training of more dental auxiliaries rather than of dentists. Again, we suggest bonuses to induce expansion for those schools with small entering classes, which would provide an incentive for expansion but would not compel it. The training of dental auxiliary personnel should also be encouraged through capitation payments, to be discussed below.

Acceleration of Medical and Dental Education

The Carnegie Commission (1970) strongly recommended acceleration of M.D. candidate education or of the total duration of premedical and medical education. The recommendation was made at a time when there was a substantial movement among medical schools in that direction. A 1970 survey indicated that 19 medical schools had started or were definitely planning to start a three-year program, while 14 schools had such a plan under consideration (Page, 1970). The movement was influenced by several interrelated considerations: (1) developments in the premedical curriculum, such as the increasing practice of requiring biochemistry for a biology or chemistry major, meant that many students entered medical school better prepared than those who had entered some years earlier; and (2) the total duration of medical education often lasted 12 to 14 years between graduation from high school and completion of specialty training—at the same time the shortage of physicians and the rapidly rising costs of medical education were widely recognized as serious problems.

While expressing a preference for a three-year M.D. candi-

[6]The Senate bill includes provisions for mandatory increases in dental-school entering classes (but not for medical schools), similar to those in the 1971 legislation, or, as an alternative for the school, the development of a Training in Expanded Auxiliary Management Program, that is, a program under which dental students are trained to treat patients with the assistance of auxiliary trained personnel.

date program, as the path to acceleration, the Carnegie Commission listed a number of different ways (1970, pp. 47-48) in which acceleration might be accomplished: (1) straightforward revision of the curriculum for M.D. candidates so that the required courses could be completed in a three-year period; (2) provisions for advanced standing for students entering with extensive premedical preparation; (3) providing instruction for M.D. candidates during all or part of the summer; (4) reducing the total number of years required for premedical and medical education combined; and (5) eliminating the free-standing internship year, a step that had already been approved by the American Medical Association in June 1970 and that became fully effective for the first time in 1974-75.

The Commission included dental education in its recommendations for acceleration but with less emphasis, because the total duration of predental and dental education has tended to be much less prolonged than that of medical education. Dental schools require only two or three years of predental education, in contrast with medical schools, which usually express a preference for candidates with B.A. degrees. In practice, however, probably under the influence of a rise in the ratio of applications to admissions, the percentage of first-year dental students who enter with a B.A. or higher degree has been growing and had reached 81 percent by 1974-75 (American Association of Dental Schools, 1975, p. 8). Although traditionally, relatively few dental-school graduates have gone on to postgraduate education, this situation is changing.

The movement toward a three-year M.D. program gained momentum in the early 1970s. It was encouraged by the provision of the 1971 health-manpower legislation that allowed $6,000 to a school for each graduate of a three-year program, compared with $4,000 for each graduate of a four-year program (see Section 2).

By 1973-74, there were 17 medical schools whose regular M.D. candidate program was three years long and 30 schools in which an optional three-year program was available (Association of American Medical Colleges, 1974, p. 44). In a few instances there had been a substantial shortening of combined premedical and medical education, either on the same campus or through cooperation between a medical school and a separate under-graduate institution. Three-year programs do not appear to have become more prevalent since 1973-74, although there have been some shifts in the practices of individual schools.[7] Optional three-year programs continue to be more prevalent than regular three-year programs. The failure of accelerated programs to spread to all medical schools appears to be attributable to opposition within some medical-school faculties and perhaps, also, to diminution of a sense of urgency about the need to shorten the duration of medical education as concern over shortages has been replaced by references to impending surpluses. But the adoption of accelerated programs has played a role in accounting for the pronounced increase in the size of entering classes and thus for the prospect of a disappearance of the shortage. A regular three-year program, and, to a more modified extent, an optional three-year program will tend to facilitate increasing the size of a school's entering class by reducing the number of student places represented by those in their fourth year of medical study. In fact, nine schools with regular three-year programs experienced, on the average, a considerably more pronounced increase in the size of their entering classes from 1968-69 to 1974-75 than the overall increase for all medical schools. (We have had to exclude from this analysis the eight schools with regular three-year programs that were relatively new and had no students in 1968-69.)

In developing our projections of the future supply of physicians, we have estimated the impact of regular and optional three-year programs on the number of graduates, but have assumed that three-year programs will not spread to many schools in the future. In this connection, it should be pointed out that a shift to three-year programs could greatly increase the number of graduates for a time, but it would gradually cease to have any effect as the proportion of students completing a three-year program leveled off, especially if the number of entrants also leveled off.

[7]We have analyzed, for example, the schools' descriptions of their curricula for 1977-78 (Association of American Medical Colleges, 1976a).

Studies of the impact of three-year programs on the performance of medical-school graduates have thus far been limited.[8] One of the earliest studies compared students who entered an optional three-year program at the University of Minnesota Medical College in 1969 and 1970 with those who opted for the four-year program. The choice between the two programs was made after the second year of medical school. Although the students opting for the three-year program tended to be somewhat older than those choosing the four-year program, the two groups did not differ significantly in academic performance on entry into medical school or during the first two years of M.D. candidate education (Garrard and Weber, 1974).

A more recent study, based on questionnaires to deans of medical schools, included replies from 14 schools with regular three-year programs and 16 schools that offered an optional three-year program. In the schools with optional programs, 22.5 percent of the students elected the three-year program, and among these students 89 percent successfully completed it. In the schools with regular three-year programs, 95 percent of the students were graduated in three years. Among 15 schools that had changed from four- to three-year programs or had optional three-year programs, there was only one in which any differences in student performance were found between those completing a four-year and those completing a three-year program. Moreover, the great majority of deans in schools with regular or optional three-year programs reported that students were pleased with the three-year program.

On the other hand, the study revealed some faculty unhappiness with acceleration. Approximately one-half of the respondents in schools with regular or optional three-year programs indicated that the faculty was not pleased with the three-year program because of time demands on both faculty members and students. A frequently cited reason for faculty dissatisfaction was the elimination of some previously taught material (Page and Boulger, 1976). There have also been some

---

[8] However, a comprehensive study of three-year curricula is now being conducted by the AAMC.

reports of student dissatisfaction with regular three-year programs that achieve acceleration by operating through part or all of the summer rather than by restructuring the curriculum. The student objections emphasize the fact that the schedule permits no relief from intensive study and provides no opportunity for the laboratory and hospital jobs that give students in four-year programs opportunities for both earning and practical experience ("Medical Course of 3 Years Tried," 1973).

There has been a substantial movement toward acceleration in dental schools as well. In fact, the proportion with some type of three-year or accelerated program is higher than among medical schools. Of the 59 dental schools, 14 offered a program that could be completed in three calendar years, while 17 had optional programs that allowed a student to complete the requirements in less than four years (American Association of Dental Schools, 1975a). However, there have been some indications recently of a reversion to four-year curricula, as the incentive of larger capitation payments has diminished.

In contrast with the 1971 legislation, the legislation now under consideration in Congress is silent on the subject of acceleration. Yet, medical education continues to be very prolonged and dental education is getting longer. We believe that opportunities should continue to be available for students to pursue a three-year program when they are qualified and motivated to undertake such a program. In fact, some medical and dental educators believe that ideally students should progress at their own pace. We suggest that this be encouraged by providing bonuses amounting to one-sixth of net educational costs to schools for each graduate completing a three-year program. The cost of such bonuses will be offset by savings in capitation payments for fourth-year students.

Detailed recommendation 3: *Additional capitation payments, designed to increase federal capitation support to about one-third of net educational costs per student should be designed to overcome geographic maldistribution of health manpower, increase enrollment in uneconomically small schools, and encourage acceleration of medical education. Schools should therefore* *qualify for payments amounting to one-sixth of net educational costs for each M.D. or D.D.S. candidate holding an NHSC scholarship, for each first-year student enrolled in a small school over and above the previous year's enrollment until first-year enrollment reaches 100;[9] and for each recipient of an M.D. or D.D.S. degree who has graduated under a three-year program.[10] Total capitation payments to any school based on M.D. or D.D.S. candidate enrollment should not exceed one-third of net educational costs per full-time student.*

Physician's Assistants and Dental Auxiliary Personnel

Programs for training physician's assistants were comparatively new and very few in number at the beginning of the 1970s, but have expanded substantially since then. The movement to train dental hygienists and dental assistants was farther advanced. Pioneering programs for training physician's assistants of varying types had been successfully initiated at Duke University, the University of Washington (Medex program), and the University of Colorado (pediatric nurse-practitioner program) in the mid- or late 1960s. By 1975, 52 programs for training physician's assistants and 2 for surgeon's assistants had been accredited by the AMA Council on Medical Education on the basis of recommendations of a joint review committee.[11]

By 1973, legislation had been enacted in a majority of the states clarifying the legal status of physician's assistants and

---

[9]To qualify for these capitation payments the school's increase in first year's enrollment would have to amount to at least 10 percent of the previous year's enrollment.

[10]When a school has a combined premedical and medical program, or a combined predental and dental program, either on one campus or in cooperation with an institution granting bachelor's degrees, permitting completion of the requirements for an M.D. or a D.D.S. degree within seven years or less following graduation from high school, capitation payments should also be provided for each graduate of such an accelerated program.

[11]The committee is composed of representatives of the American Academy of Family Physicians, American Academy of Pediatrics, American Academy of Physician's Assistants, American College of Physicians, American College of Surgeons, and American Society of Internal Medicine ("Physician's Aid Review Bodies Merge," 1975).

generally permitting them to treat patients under the supervision of an M.D. (Spingarn, 1973). The provisions differ substantially from state to state, however, and, according to Lee and others (1976), tend to limit the potential role of nurse practitioners and physician's assistants.

By the spring of 1976, an estimated 2,800 physician's assistants (including nurse practitioners) were practicing in the United States and 5,700 more were expected to graduate by the end of 1977. According to the president of the American Academy of Physician's Assistants, "they can handle about 75 percent of the common problems seen in family practice . . . ." He also indicated that studies showed "excellent patient acceptance of physician's assistants," but something of a problem with physician acceptance. However that may be, he was quoted as stating in addition that "every program has two job offers per graduate" ("Doctors Are Slow to Accept . . . ," 1976).

There is also evidence that these physician extenders are beginning to alleviate the geographic maldistribution of physicians. Medex programs, in particular (a type of physician's assistant training program that combines institutional and on-the-job training over a 12- to 24-month period), are making an impressive contribution to overcoming shortages in rural areas. A follow-up study of graduates of the nine Medex programs that had been developed by 1975 indicated that 56 percent were practicing in towns with a population of less than 10,000 and another 14 percent were in towns with populations ranging from 10,000 to 20,000. Along with this pattern of location, 76 percent were assisting physicians in general practice or family practice (general practitioners, in particular, tend to be located in small communities). The success of these programs in locating their graduates in small towns is attributed to their pattern of placing their trainees in preceptorships (on-the-job training assisting a practicing physician) in such communities. Preliminary studies of samples of graduates of two-year physician's assistant and nurse-practitioner programs, on the other hand, indicate that approximately 50 percent are employed in institutional and large-group settings, predominantly in urban and suburban areas (Lawrence, Wilson, and Castle, 1975). However, there is evidence that nurse practitioners trained in the Colorado program are practicing in rural areas of the state, and the Canadian provinces of British Columbia and Alberta rely heavily and successfully on nurse practitioners in rural areas. It is unreasonable to measure the success of programs solely in terms of their contribution to overcoming shortages in rural areas and small towns. There are severe shortages in inner-city areas as well, and some programs, such as the Medex program at Howard University, are particularly well situated to meeting such shortages.

Physician's assistant programs are costly, because their requirements in terms of faculty time and equipment are similar to those of M.D. candidate programs. Costs per student of the physician's assistant program at Duke University have been reported to be very similar to those of its M.D. candidate program (Estes and Howard, 1970). Costs of Medex programs are probably somewhat lower, because of their greater emphasis on preceptorships. Average educational costs for a nurse-practitioner program have been estimated at about $4,000 a year, with a range from $1,500 to $9,000 (Lee and others, 1976).[12] The growth of these programs can be explained to a considerable degree by federal government support, and their future growth would be jeopardized if that support were withdrawn. Early in 1975 it was reported that the Medex program at Dartmouth College, which had produced about 125 physician's assistants, was planning to close down because of reductions in federal support and the inability of the federal government to fund the program on other than a year-to-year basis ("Dartmouth to Drop . . . ," 1975).

Dental hygienist and dental assistant programs are also costly because of similar needs for close supervision and expensive equipment. However, these programs are conducted, evidently successfully, in comprehensive colleges and community colleges, where they have access to vocational education funds, as well as in dental schools. The official positions of both the

---

[12]According to the same source, annual costs of training a physician's assistant average $6,000, with a range from $2,000 to $12,000.

American Medical Association and the Association of American Medical Colleges are that physician's assistant programs should be conducted in close relationship to the training of physicians. We share that view and also believe that there is a strong case for support of some dental hygienist and dental assistant training programs in dental schools, because programs that are conducted under close supervision of dental-school faculties can serve as models for programs in other types of educational institutions. Enrollment in programs training dental auxiliary personnel has grown steadily and in 1974 totaled about 21,000, but only about one-half of existing dental schools have such programs.

The 1971 health-manpower legislation provided for capitation payments of $1,000 to medical and dental schools for each student in a physician's assistant or dental therapist training program. Current legislative proposals provide instead for special-project grants or contracts to support such programs. We believe that special-project grants are desirable for developing new programs, but that ongoing programs that meet the requirements applicable to new programs should be assured of capitation payments without having to go through the process of negotiating special-project grants or contracts periodically. Special-project grants or contracts should cover costs associated with development of the programs plus a capitation payment of $1,000 per year for each full-time enrolled student, while ongoing projects should also receive capitation payments of $1,000.

Detailed recommendation 4: *Schools should be eligible for capitation payments of $1,000 for each student enrolled in a physician's assistant, nurse-practitioner, or dental auxiliary program.*

Graduate Medical Education

The 1971 health-manpower legislation, as we have seen, included provisions for capitation payments of $3,000 for each trainee in a graduate training program in primary care (see Section 2). The capitation payments were also provided for graduate training in primary-care dentistry. We have earlier commented on the probable role of these provisions in the pronounced rise in the relative importance of primary-care residencies.

The legislative proposals now before Congress go much farther toward imposing a detailed and extensive set of controls on medical residency programs. Provisions of the Senate bill, for example, include:

1. Making capitation payments to schools of medicine and osteopathy conditional on a requirement that a stipulated and rising proportion of the school's filled residencies be in family practice, primary internal medicine, primary pediatrics, and primary obstetrics and gynecology—specifically, 42 percent in 1977-78, 47 percent in 1978-79, and 57 percent in 1979-80, with not more than 7 percent to be in obstetrics and gynecology in each of these years. These requirements are in addition to the provisions relating to the proportion of students holding NHSC scholarships, discussed earlier. Like those requirements, the residency requirements will not be enforced against individual schools if the aggregate national goals are substantially met. Alternatively, the school will not be subject to these requirements if it is complying with specific certification requirements imposed by the Secretary of HEW.
2. Special-project grants to encourage training programs in primary internal medicine and primary pediatrics, as well as in primary dental care, along the lines of provisions in the 1971 legislation, but no provision for capitation payments of $3,000 for each trainee.
3. Establishment of a National Council on Postgraduate Physician Training of 24 members to (1) sponsor studies of physician specialty distribution, (2) cooperate with each physician specialty organization to assist its activities with respect to the number and location of practitioners within each such specialty, (3) assess needs for financial support of postgraduate training and the role of postgraduate physician trainees in meeting service needs of hospitals, etc., and (4) assess the impact of the medical service of FMGs in the United States.

4. Establishment of 10 regional councils on postgraduate physician training of 24 members each, with responsibilities within each region similar to those set forth for the National Council on a nationwide basis.

5. Determination by the Secretary of HEW, in accordance with the recommendations of the National Council, of the total number of postgraduate physician-training positions to be certified for each fiscal year, beginning with 1978-79. The number of first-year residencies may not exceed 110 percent of the number of M.D.s expected to be granted in the United States in any year, except that transitional provisions for 1978-79 and 1979-80 call for 140 and 125 percent, respectively, of the number of U.S. medical graduates.[13]

6. Determination, within this overall number, of the number of positions in each specialty or subspecialty (taking into consideration the findings of studies sponsored by the National Council), and the number of such specialty or subspecialty positions to be assigned within each of the 10 regions. Exceptions may be made, to the extent of not more than 10 percent of the total number of positions, for specialties in which the national need for positions is not sufficient to permit regional allocation.

7. Certification by the Secretary, on the recommendation of each regional council, of postgraduate physician-training positions in entities that directly provide such training within each region. These certifications may not exceed the total number authorized for the region and should aim at equitable geographic distribution within the region and the maintenance of acceptable educational standards.

8. Termination of financial assistance of all types to any entity maintaining a postgraduate physician-training position that is not certified in accordance with these provisions. Entities will also be subject to civil penalties for maintaining such positions.

[13]A similar provision in H.R. 5546 (House version) was defeated on the floor of the House by a vote of 207 to 146 ("Service by Health Students," 1975). The Senate also acted early in July 1976 (as this report was being printed) to delete HEW residency controls.

These provisions add up to a set of federal controls on physician residency programs that are not paralleled by controls in any other field. Granted that the controls are designed to limit the participation of FMGs in residency programs, and to achieve improved geographic and specialty distribution, it is highly questionable whether such an elaborate set of federal controls is the best means of achieving the desired objectives. We have noted that the proportion of residents in primary-care training has increased substantially in recent years under federal provisions that have provided financial support for family-practice programs, capitation payments for residents in primary-care programs, state support for family-practice programs, and other influences. We have also shown that the proportion of FMGs among residents has begun to decline (Figure 3). (We shall have more to say about appropriate restrictions on FMGs at a later point.)

Not previously discussed in this connection is the establishment (in 1972) of the Liaison Committee on Graduate Medical Education with the intention that it would become the official accrediting body for graduate medical education, paralleling the role of the Liaison Committee on Medical Education, which has existed since 1942 as the official accrediting body for undergraduate medical education. The Liaison Committee on Graduate Medical Education is sponsored by five parent organizations —the American Medical Association, American Board of Medical Specialties, Association of American Medical Colleges, American Hospital Association, and Council of Medical Specialty Societies. Formerly all accreditation decisions relating to residencies were made independently by 23 separate residency review committees ("Medical Education in the United States, 1974-75," 1975, p. 1326).

It is too early to determine what the impact of the liaison committee will be, because it did not begin its official function as an accrediting body until early in 1975. Moreover, it will continue to receive recommendations from the residency review committees, which will therefore continue to have considerable influence on the accreditation process. The Coordinating Council on Medical Education (CCME), which is sponsored by the same five organizations as the liaison committee, plays an important role in overseeing the policies of the liaison committee. Although the coordinating council has endorsed a goal of 50 percent of all residencies in primary-care training, it does not attempt to control the number of residencies in any specialty except insofar as it considers such factors as the relationship of the size of the faculty to the number of trainees in a given program (Holden and others, 1976, p. 1429).

Some medical experts who do not support the strict controls over residencies that have been included in recent congressional proposals nevertheless believe that the federal government should establish an overall limit on the number of residencies. Among these experts is Dr. Philip R. Lee, who favors an overall limit of 125 percent of U.S. medical graduates by 1980, with enforcement by the Secretary of HEW, preferably in cooperation with the CCME, but with the Secretary having final authority. He also favors a requirement that 50 percent of all residencies (not including obstetrics/gynecology) be in primary-care training and feels that the federal government, which already exerts substantial influence through its policies for reimbursement of hospital and patient-care costs in the Medicare and Medicaid programs, should refrain from reimbursing hospitals for residencies considered excessive, for example, surgical residencies and subspecialty residencies in various fields (Lee, 1976, p. 1686).

The AAMC also favors federal controls that are not as far-reaching as those included in some recent congressional proposals.[14]

A relatively modest provision would be the establishment of an overall ceiling on residencies without detailed control of regional and specialty distribution or of the number provided by individual entities. However, apart from the question as to how such an overall ceiling could be enforced without detailed controls, there remains a substantial question as to whether it will be necessary if the inflow of FMGs is restricted, as seems virtually certain. Enforcement of a ceiling tied by formula to

[14]These provisions are included in S. 992, March 6, 1975, which was introduced by Senator Kennedy on behalf of the AAMC.

the number of U.S. medical graduates could result in excessive rigidity in a situation in which flexible adaptation to future needs is desirable. We have seen that the adoption of a comprehensive national health-insurance system could result in a significant increase in the demand for physicians' services. Adaptation to such an increase in demand—especially in view of the geographic disparities in supply of health manpower—could be impaired by a strict ceiling on the number of residents and thus could exacerbate the inflation in health-care costs that would be likely to result from adoption of national health insurance.

In addition to the concern over FMGs, and their uneven geographic distribution, a major objective of those who support residency controls is to increase the proportion of residencies in primary-care training. We have seen that changes in the desired direction are under way and believe that they should continue to be encouraged by policies that emphasize incentives rather than by compulsion. Along with provisions for special-project grants to encourage postgraduate primary-care training in both medicine and dentistry, we favor capitation grants to schools and hospitals amounting to $3,000 for each trainee in a primary-care program over and above the number in the immediately preceding year. With the change that is already under way in the specialty distribution of first-year residents, the need for such a provision might well disappear by the early 1980s.

Reimbursement policies under federal Medicare and Medicaid programs also need to be modified. According to a special report prepared by the Institute of Medicine of the National Academy of Sciences, "Medicare and Medicaid payments support faculty and house officer salaries in teaching hospitals, and would seem to favor the present pattern of the education process—greater specialization—over the establishment of new training—ambulatory care—because of less favorable reimbursement provisions for outpatient care" (U.S. House of Representatives, 1976, p. 9). Prevailing charges tend to be higher in areas with high physician-population ratios and in high-income areas and large metropolitan areas generally.[15]

[15] For an extensive discussion of problems associated with reimbursement policies, see Lee and others (1976).

The report made a number of recommendations designed to meet these problems, including: (1) a change in financing mechanisms to provide more equitable support for ambulatory care services; (2) direct support to medical schools and teaching hospitals through special-project grants for the support of primary-care training; (3) monitoring of the specialty distribution of physicians and the number of residency slots by a quasi-public independent physician-manpower commission, with enforcement of its determinations to be the responsibility of the Liaison Committee on Graduate Medical Education for a three-year period, after which the legislative authority for the Secretary of HEW might be sought if the commission's determinations have not been implemented;[16] (4) interim freezing of the number of specialty training slots (other than in family practice, general internal medicine, and general pediatrics) until recommendation 3 is implemented; (5) a major study of the basis of physician fees and fee allowances in public and private health-insurance programs; (6) discontinuance of Medicaid practices that pay physicians less in one geographic area than in another; and (7) a detailed examination of Medicaid administrative practices to determine the extent to which these practices affect the availability of physician services in underserved areas.

Some of the issues raised by these recommendations are complex, especially in view of the role of the states in determining Medicaid policies. Because they are concerned with the impact of provisions under the Social Security Act rather than directly with health-manpower education policies, they are to some degree beyond the purview of the Carnegie Council. Nevertheless, the important point is that existing policies do run counter to attempts to overcome overspecialization and geographic disparities and, to the extent feasible, should be changed.

Detailed recommendation 5: *Special-project grants to encourage the development of family practice and primary dental-care*

[16]The responsibility of the liaison committee would be shared by the CCME and the American Osteopathic Committee on Postdoctoral Training.

training programs should be continued, and capitation grants of $3,000 for each resident in a primary-care training program (family practice, primary internal medicine, primary pediatrics, primary obstetrics and gynecology, and primary dentistry) over and above the number in such training programs in the preceding year should be provided.

Congress should give serious consideration to the recommendations of the Institute of Medicine of the National Academy of Sciences for changes in reimbursement policies under Medicare and Medicaid, but strict federal controls on residencies should be avoided.

Foreign Medical Graduates

There is a reasonable probability that the inflow of FMGs will decline as the supply of U.S. medical graduates increases. Granted that inferior opportunities for medical graduates in some of the countries of emigration, such as the Philippines, may tend to "push" FMGs toward this country, they are much less likely to come, and even more unlikely to remain, as the strength of the "pull" force, that is, of shortages of medical manpower, in this country diminishes. Immigration, even of highly educated manpower, has always been responsive to changes in economic conditions. And, in fact, the percentage of FMGs among interns and residents declined in 1973-74 (Figure 3).

Nevertheless, certain changes in policy are needed to limit the inflow of FMGs, especially those with inferior qualifications. Immigration of FMGs has been encouraged by the Immigration and Nationalization Act amendments of 1965.[17] Termination of the national-origins quota system opened the door, which had previously been largely closed, to immigration from Asia and other parts of the world that had not traditionally supplied many immigrants. In addition, preferential immigration status was assigned to persons with professional and occupational skills deemed to be in short supply, as determined by the Department of Labor. Physicians were ruled to be one of these

[17]Public Law 89-236, October 3, 1965.

occupations by the Department in 1965. In view of the rapidly increasing supply of U.S. medical graduates, this preferred status should now be removed.

In addition, FMGs need to meet standards of admission to residency programs that are as closely comparable as possible with those met by U.S. medical graduates, as a 1974 task force of the AAMC recommended ("Graduates of Foreign Medical Schools . . . ," 1974). Since 1958, the Educational Commission for Foreign Medical Graduates (ECFMG) has been responsible for administering a special examination to FMGs applying for visas through a worldwide network of 178 examination centers.[18] The examination consists largely of questions taken from Part II of the National Board of Medical Examiners examination.

Health manpower legislative proposals now before Congress would amend the Immigration and Nationalization Act to tighten provisions relating to entry of FMGs and to require that they have passed Parts I and II of the National Board of Medical Examiners examination before being admitted to a residency program in the United States. They would also be required to demonstrate adequate knowledge of English. We believe that these amendments are desirable.

Detailed recommendation 6: *Foreign medical graduates should be required to meet the same standards as U.S. medical graduates for admission to residency programs, and immigration legislation and regulations should be amended to remove preferential immigration status for physicians.*

Standards for State Licensure

Partly related to the FMG problem are provisions in current legislative proposals requiring the Secretary of HEW to develop, in consultation with appropriate organizations, model standards for state licensure of physicians and dentists. Quite apart from the FMG problem, such standards have long been needed to

---

[18]The ECFMG is sponsored by the AAMC, American Hospital Association, Association for Hospital Medical Education, American Medical Association, and Federation of State Medical Boards.

bring about greater uniformity in licensing requirements among the states. We support these proposals.[19]

Detailed recommendation 7: *The Secretary of Health, Education, and Welfare should be charged with the responsibility of developing national standards for state licensing of physicians and dentists, and state licensing agencies should enforce licensing requirements for all foreign medical graduates employed within each state.*

Special-Project Grants

Although we place major emphasis on capitation payments to provide basic federal support to medical and dental schools and to induce desired policy changes, there are certain purposes for which special-project grants are more appropriate. We believe that health-manpower legislation should include provision for special-project grants for (1) development of new programs for training physician's assistants, nurse practitioners, and dental auxiliaries, (2) development of new programs for training in family medicine and primary dental care, (3) educational assistance for individuals from disadvantaged backgrounds, (4) educational assistance or special educational programs for U.S. citizens who have been enrolled in foreign medical schools, (5) development of area health education programs (to be discussed fully in Section 7), and (6) curriculum innovation and reform.

A number of states have provided funds for decentralization of clinical training and for the development of family practice or, more generally, primary-care residency programs. We believe that the federal government should encourage other

[19]One of the recommendations of the Carnegie Commission (1970, p. 78) called for the appointment of a National Health Manpower Commission, which, among other things, would investigate the feasibility of national licensing requirements for all health manpower. Also pertinent is the recommendation of the 1974 AAMC task force that steps be taken by the Federation of State Medical Boards to enforce licensing requirements for the substantial numbers of FMGs who are delivering medical services in state institutions and other medical-service organizations on the basis of temporary licenses or exemptions from licensing provisions ("Graduates of Foreign Medical Schools . . . ," 1974).

states to take similar action by making a portion of the funds appropriated for special-project grants available for matching grants to states at the discretion of the Secretary of HEW.

In view of the indications—to be discussed in Section 6—that we are developing too many new medical schools, we are opposed to start-up grants or other types of grants to support the development of innovative medical schools, medical schools especially designed to train students for practice in ambulatory-care settings, regional health-professions schools (to the extent that they would be involved in M.D. candidate programs), or other similar proposals that have been included in bills recently under consideration. There should be continuing provision for start-up grants sufficient to meet the needs of the relatively few new schools that we suggest in Section 6, and for developing schools designed to encourage members of minority groups. There should also be continuing provisions for construction grants and loans to meet the needs of these few new schools and of necessary renovation or reconstruction at existing schools.

This does not mean that we are opposed to innovation in medical schools, training for ambulatory-care settings, or other objectives contemplated by these provisions. But we see no reason why such programs cannot be developed within existing medical schools and, for some of the clinical training involved, in area health education centers.

In Section 1, we have mentioned the impressive progress in curriculum reform, with particular reference to early clinical experience for medical students and integration of basic science and clinical science components of the curriculum. Despite the progress that has been made, such changes continue to need encouragement, and some dental educators consider that they have not proceeded nearly far enough in dental-school curricula.

Sharp criticism of both dental education and the dental profession was made at an AADS meeting in the spring of 1975 (Watkins, 1975). Dean Sheldon Rovin of the University of Washington School of Dentistry advocates a thoroughgoing set of changes in dental education aimed at greater emphasis on primary care that would include especially: changing the admissions process to attract those most qualified for primary care; moving the basic sciences into the predental curriculum; substantially increasing the amount of behavioral science in the dental curriculum; more curriculum emphasis on diagnosis; initiating student group practices as the vehicle for patient care; emphasis on intra- and interdisciplinary training; extending the curriculum;[20] establishing general practice or primary-care residencies; making more rational use of existing auxiliaries, with the eventual goal of auxiliaries performing most of the routine functions; and ultimately integrating dentistry into medicine so that the future primary-care practitioner receives both medical and dental training (Rovin, 1976).

Continuing provision for "financial distress" grants should be designed merely to phase out existing grants of this type.

Detailed recommendation 8: *Provision should be made for special-project grants for (1) development of new programs for training physician's assistants, nurse practitioners, and dental auxiliaries, (2) development of new programs for training in family medicine and primary dental care, (3) educational assistance for individuals from disadvantaged backgrounds, (4) educational assistance or special educational programs for U.S. citizens who have been enrolled in foreign medical schools, (5) development of area health education centers, and (6) curriculum innovation and reform.*

At the discretion of the Secretary of HEW, some of the special-project grants should be awarded to state governments on a matching fund basis.

Tuition Controls

Legislative proposals include a provision requiring the Secretary of HEW to establish criteria for determining allowable increases in tuition and other educational costs. The requirement is

---

[20]He is not opposed to acceleration of dental education, which should encourage progress of the student at his own pace, but he considers adequate training for primary care to require a longer curriculum for the average student (letter to Clark Kerr, June 21, 1976).

related to the greatly increased role of NHSC scholarships contemplated under these proposals and the fact that tuition and
other educational costs are covered by the scholarships. Also
involved are direct student loans, which may not exceed the
cost of tuition plus $2,500.

In view of the role the states play in determining the tuition policy of their public medical and dental schools, and their
increasing role in providing funds for private medical and dental
schools (see Section 8), intrusion of the federal government into
tuition decisions is questionable. At the same time, the fact that
tuition will be fully covered by federal funds for a substantial
proportion of students does give rise to a possibility that some
health-professions schools may take advantage of the situation
to impose sharp tuition increases. We believe, however, that the
federal government should not become involved in determining
allowable increases in tuition in health science centers with their
highly complex problems of determining true net educational
costs.[21]

Detailed recommendation 9: *Federal government involvement
in determining allowable tuition increases of medical and dental
schools should be avoided.*

---

[21]For a detailed analysis of the factors associated with wide variations
among the states in tuition charges of public institutions of higher education and the difficulties that would arise from federal policies designed to
encourage low or no tuition in the first two years of college, see Carnegie
Council (1975a).

5

The National Health Service Corps and Student Assistance

Geographic maldistribution of health manpower can be overcome only by a combination of policies, as we have suggested earlier; among these policies, expansion of the National Health Service Corps and the related scholarship program should play an important role. There are several reasons for this:

1. The needs of underserved areas are unlikely to be adequately met, despite appropriate combinations of other policies, by movements of private practitioners into those areas.
2. Geographic allocation of NHSC personnel can be shifted in accordance with changing needs in a manner that would not be feasible for private practitioners.
3. NHSC employment provides valuable initial professional experience for young physicians and dentists (along with other health personnel) in circumstances that enhance their understanding of relationships between economic deprivation and poor health.
4. Members of the NHSC may elect to practice in communities in which they have served, having established a potential clientele among patients served through the corps. It is too early to have much evidence on this point, but it is encour-

aging that in the last three years the percentage of physicians electing to continue their NHSC service beyond the initial period has increased from 3 to 30 percent (Lee and others, 1976).

Establishment of the Corps

The National Health Service Corps (NHSC) was established under provisions of the Emergency Health Personnel Act of 1970.[1] In view of the long history of opposition from the American Medical Association (AMA) and from other groups to anything that might open the door to "socialized medicine," supporters of the legislation felt considerable apprehension over its chances of enactment, but their efforts were successful, and the leading congressional supporters of the bill managed to forestall a threatened presidential veto ("The Dance of Legislation . . . ," 1974). In fact, the AMA has consistently supported the NHSC, while showing particular support for policies that require periodic review of the need for corps members in any given area (Nesbitt and Ruhe, 1975, p. 509).

The legislation authorized establishment within the U.S. Public Health Service of an administrative unit to improve the delivery of health services to underserved communities and areas. Personnel were to be assigned to areas designed by the Secretary of HEW as having critical health-manpower shortages, but only upon request of a state or local health agency or other public or nonprofit private health organization. The need also had to be certified by district medical or dental societies and by the local government of the area. Persons receiving services were to be charged at rates established by the Secretary, but provisions could be made for furnishing the service at reduced rates or without charge for persons determined to be unable to pay full charges. Health facilities of the area were to be utilized, but when they were lacking, facilities could be leased or otherwise provided or the nearest health facilities of the U.S. Public Health Service could be utilized. Establishment of the National

[1] Public Law 91-623, December 31, 1970.

Advisory Council on Health Manpower Shortages was also authorized.[2]

Appropriations for the NHSC have been modest—amounting to about $12 to $14 million in the last few years—and the size of the corps has grown slowly. From an initial placement of 20 health professionals in 16 communities, the corps had expanded by 1975 to include 551 professionals serving communities in 40 states (*Supplemental Appropriations . . .* , 1975, p. 1067). Corps physicians were receiving salaries of about $12,000 a year, but bonuses, it was reported, brought their compensation up to $28,000 (Hicks, 1974).

On the whole, the available evidence indicates that the corps has been effective and that support for it has grown within the Administration, Congress, and in professional health-manpower circles. Health-manpower legislative proposals now before Congress provide for authorizations substantially larger than funds that have been made available previously. Under H.R. 5546 (House version), the authorization would rise from $30 to $45 million between fiscal year 1976 and 1978, while under the Senate version of the bill it would rise from $47 to $70 million over a three-year period beginning in fiscal 1978.

The services of an expanded Corps would unquestionably be utilized. In 1975, 1,128 communities had been designated as eligible, and 445 had been approved. Substantial progress has also been made in matching assignments of corpsmen to communities for which they have expressed a preference. Opposition of local medical societies is reported to have been relatively rare, although opposition of local dental societies has appar-

---

[2] A few modifications of the original legislation were made under the Emergency Health Personnel Act Amendments of 1972 (Public Law 92-585, October 27, 1972). Among the more important of these was a provision that the Secretary could disregard opposition of state or district medical or dental societies, if the need had been certified by the other appropriate state and local bodies and if he or she found that certification of the local professional societies had been "arbitrarily and capriciously withheld." Also added was a provision for collection of payments from public or other third-party agencies that would have been responsible for providing the care in the absence of health corps services.

ently been somewhat more frequent (*Supplemental Appropriations . . .* , 1975, p. 1067).

The bills now before Congress include more extensive provisions relating to the NHSC than did the acts of 1970 and 1972. There are more detailed criteria for the designation of health-manpower shortage areas, including consideration of such factors as infant mortality rates and the employment of FMGs in the area, as well as ratios of health manpower to population. The Senate version also calls for giving special consideration to applications from entities that will utilize physician's assistants, nurse practitioners, or expanded-function dental auxiliaries to assist corps members.

The House version includes a provision specifically designed to make the compensation of physician and dentist corps members competitive with that of individuals in private practice. Under this provision the Secretary of HEW is authorized to increase the member's monthly pay and allowance by an amount (not to exceed $1,000) that will provide "a monthly income competitive with the average monthly income from a practice of an individual" in the same profession with equivalent training and experience.

NHSC Scholarships

The NHSC scholarship program is designed to strengthen recruitment to the corps and, under current legislative proposals, would be by far the most important grant program for health-professions students. It was established under legislation adopted in 1972, which authorized the Secretary of HEW to establish the Public Health and National Health Service Corps Scholarship Training Program "to obtain trained physicians, dentists, nurses, and other health-related specialists for the National Health Service Corps and other units of the Service."[3] To be eligible, an individual had to be enrolled (or accepted for enrollment) as a full-time student in a program leading to a degree in medicine, dentistry, or other health-related specialty,

[3] Public Law 92-585, October 27, 1972.

as determined by the Secretary, and also had to be eligible for appointment to the corps.

Each participant would receive an annual scholarship during each year of training (not to exceed four years) that would include tuition, other necessary educational expenses, and an amount not to exceed the basic pay and allowances of a commissioned officer on active duty, in pay grade O-1 with less than two years of service.[4] In return, the recipient would be obligated to serve as a commissioned officer in the Public Health Service or as a civilian member of the NHSC following completion of his or her academic training, on a basis of one year of service for each year during which he or she had received the scholarship. The required service could follow internship and residency years in the case of physicians and dentists. However, periods of internship and residency would be creditable toward the service obligation if served in a facility of the Public Health Service or of the NHSC.

Failure to complete all or any part of the period of required service would entail an obligation to repay scholarship funds received plus interest (for an equivalent period) to the federal government within three years. Failure to complete an academic program would entail a similar obligation.

The initial legislation authorized $3 million for fiscal 1974, but an appropriation of $22.5 million was made available for fiscal 1975. H.R. 5546 (House version) authorizes amounts increasing from $40 million for fiscal 1976 to $120 million for fiscal 1978, while the Senate version calls for amounts rising from $85 million in fiscal 1978 to $233 million in fiscal 1980. The Senate version also earmarks about 95 percent of the funds for scholarships to medical, osteopathic, or dental students.

Both bills stiffen the repayment obligation by calling for repayments amounting to double, or triple (in the Senate bill) the scholarship funds received plus interest, while the Senate version calls for such payment within 60 days of the date of breach of contract.

[4]The Secretary was authorized to arrange to pay tuition and other educational expenses directly to the institution.

On the other hand, the service obligation is made somewhat more flexible under provisions that permit the Secretary to release an individual from service in the corps on the basis of a written agreement to enter private practice in an underserved area. The individual must agree to charge the prevailing fees for service in the area, provide services at reduced fees or no fees for persons unable to pay prevailing charges, and not discriminate against Medicare or Medicaid recipients.[5]

What has been the experience thus far with NHSC scholarships? From the beginning, the number of applicants has substantially exceeded the number of scholarships available. In 1974-75, 1,480 scholarships were awarded, averaging about $10,000 a year for tuition, fees, and living expenses ("1,480 Scholarships Awarded . . . ," 1975). In the following year, 895 scholarships were awarded, bringing the total since the beginning of the program to 2,745 ("HEW Awarded . . . ," 1976). In announcing the scholarships, the Bureau of Health Manpower indicated that preference would be given to students on the basis of interest in primary-care training, academic performance, and nearness to graduation. Secondary factors would be commitment to enter primary-care practice in a health-manpower shortage area, work experience in medically underserved areas, and residence in such areas ("HEW Mails . . . ," 1975).

The authorizations in the Senate bill now under consideration contemplate bringing the total number of NHSC scholarship holders up to approximately one-third of medical students and one-fifth of dental students—proportions commensurate with the proportion of students the schools would be required to admit. This would mean some 18,000 to 19,000 medical students and about 4,000 dental students.[6]

---

[5]The House version also includes provisions for grants to assist such individuals in getting started in private practice and for subsidies to compensate them for deficiencies in their incomes below what they would have earned in the corps, but the Senate version does not include comparable provisions.

[6]Total enrollment of M.D. candidates in medical schools in 1974-75 was about 54,100, while enrollment of D.D.S. candidates in dental schools was about 20,100. In addition, total enrollment in schools of osteopathy may be estimated at close to 3,000.

Experience with the much smaller numbers of NHSC scholarships available thus far does not shed much light on whether there would be enough qualified applicants for the much larger number of scholarships contemplated in the future. However, as we noted in Section 4, the scholarships are generous, and the compensation of those who serve in the corps is deliberately designed to be competitive with compensation in private practice. This is likely to be an increasingly attractive feature as the supply of U.S. medical graduates increases and competition for promising openings in relatively well-served areas intensifies.

In this connection, the experience with forgiveness features in loan programs needs to be mentioned. It will be recalled (Section 2) that federal provisions for loans to students in the health professions include forgiveness features for those who practice in underserved areas (either in the NHSC or in private practice). The amounts forgiven are by no means negligible—30 percent of outstanding principal and interest after one year of practice in an underserved area, another 30 percent after two years, and an additional 25 percent after three years.[7] Even so, a General Accounting Office study showed that, by October 1973, among approximately 30,000 medical and dental students who had received loans from 1965 to 1972, only a tiny fraction (well under 1 percent) had taken advantage of the loan forgiveness option, and most of these would have located in a shortage area without the inducement of loan forgiveness (Comptroller General, 1974, p. 40). A number of states have had loan programs with similar forgiveness features, and follow-up studies have again shown the impact on the location of physicians to have been negligible.

Why, then, should the NHSC scholarship provisions be expected to be more effective in inducing location in underserved areas? There is little experience to go on thus far, but the federal loan program calls for repayment over a ten-year period

---

[7] Loan forgiveness features, though considerably less liberal than these, were included in the Health Professions Educational Assistance Amendments of 1965.

following completion of medical or dental training (including internship and residency and any period of military service). Thus annual repayments are not likely to represent a sizable proportion of professional earnings unless the outstanding indebtedness is very large. NHSC provisions, however, call for repayment of scholarship funds within three years on failure to honor the commitment to serve in an underserved area (the Senate bill would call for repayment within 60 days, as we have seen). In addition, the total repayment burden, especially for an individual who had received an NHSC scholarship for four years, could well run to $50,000 or more (without the proposed double- or triple-obligation feature).

We strongly support the proposed expansion of both the NHSC and the NHSC scholarship program, while refraining from detailed comment on certain features of the proposals that are not entirely acceptable to some of those who support the programs. In particular, we are not convinced that double- or triple-repayment provisions are essential to achieving compliance with the commitment to serve in underserved areas. And, along with Lee and others (1976), we believe that a two-year service commitment might be preferable to the four years that would be required for a student who received an NHSC scholarship program for four years. In fact, there is at least a possibility that excessive requirements and penalties could deter voluntary signing up for the program.

Other Student Assistance

Current legislative proposals involve significant changes in existing student aid provisions. The House bill would phase out the scholarship program for needy students, allowing only for continuing awards to students already holding grants, while the Senate bill includes a modest provision for scholarships to students of exceptional financial need in their first year of postbaccalaureate study in schools of medicine, osteopathy, dentistry, and other specific health-professions schools.

We believe that there is a case for a scholarship program of modest proportions with emphasis on, but not limited to, first-year students, to encourage enrollment of students from disadvantaged backgrounds without forcing them into the NHSC scholarship program. This is not to deny the desirability of maximum emphasis on the NHSC program, but simply to recognize that students from middle- and upper-income families are in a better position to finance their postbaccalaureate education with only limited borrowing if they wish to avoid the commitment associated with an NHSC scholarship than are students from disadvantaged backgrounds. Students from disadvantaged backgrounds tend to be highly conscious of their extremely limited family assets and to be wary of the very substantial borrowing that is often required to finance medical or dental education.

Despite the encouraging rise in the proportions of medical and dental students from minority-group backgrounds in recent years, it will be a long time before the extremely small percentages of minority-group members among practicing physicians and dentists are appreciably increased.

Important changes are also made in loan provisions, generally tending to de-emphasize the existing direct student loan program and establishing a new program of federally insured loans for health-professions students. Among other things, the interest rate on direct student loans is raised from 3 to 7 percent. There is considerable concern about this change on the part of health-professions educators, but the 3 percent interest rate in student loan programs dates from the National Defense Education Act of 1958, when interest rates were far below their present levels, and there is an inequity between those who can receive direct loans at 3 percent and those who must pay 7 percent for guaranteed loans under current provisions of the Higher Education Act.

In its report *The Federal Role in Postsecondary Education* (1975b, pp. 42-47), the Carnegie Council pointed out serious inadequacies and inequities in existing federal loan programs. These problems would be perpetuated for health professions students under the proposed provisions. In our 1975 report, we recommended the phasing out of existing loan programs and their replacement by a National Student Loan Bank. Because of the relatively heavy reliance of medical and dental students on loans as a means of financing, the establishment of such a bank would be especially advantageous for them.[8]

Among the major weaknesses of the guaranteed loan program discussed in our 1975 report are the following:

1. A basic problem of inequality of opportunity in a program in which lenders, and especially bank lenders, are likely to be influenced by the credit standing of the student's family and probably, also, by the family's socioeconomic status in the community
2. The difficulty of ensuring student access to loans in a tight money market
3. The lack of incentive for banks and other lenders to pursue adequate collection procedures when loans are guaranteed by the federal government
4. A fundamental question as to whether interest subsidies, as opposed to deferral of interest during periods of enrollment, are appropriate
5. The disadvantages of a short period of repayment—difficult to avoid when banks predominate among the lenders—in view of the life-cycle in income and expenditures (Carnegie Council, 1975b, pp. 43-45).

The National Student Loan Bank would be a nonprofit private corporation chartered by the federal government and financed by the sale of government-guaranteed securities. There would be reasonable limits on the amounts that could be borrowed, and borrowers would repay loans by paying approximately three-fourths of 1 percent of income each year for each $1,000 borrowed until the total loan and accrued interest was

[8]Medical and dental students are particularly dependent on loans for a number of reasons: the costs of medical and dental education are high; they are past the age when parents typically expect to provide for educational expenses; and part-time employment of students during the academic year is not very feasible (and is often discouraged by schools) because of lengthy instructional and laboratory periods and study requirements. For recent data on borrowing by medical and dental students, see "Medical Education in the United States, 1974-75" (1975, p. 1345) and American Dental Association (1975, p. 17).

repaid. Thus, repayments would be related to income, but the program would not involve redistribution of income, as would proposals for an Economic Opportunity Bank. Rather, it would involve varying numbers of years for repayment, depending on the income level of the debtor. The average income earner would require about 20 years for repayment.[9] The successful experience of the Student Loan Marketing Association (Sallie Mae) suggests that it could be restructured into a National Student Loan Bank and that both private and public funds could be involved.

Detailed recommendation 10: *The Council recommends expanded federal financial support for the National Health Service Corps and the associated NHSC scholarship program, along the lines of current legislative proposals. In addition to the NHSC scholarship program, the Council recommends a scholarship program for medical and dental students of exceptional financial need, with major emphasis on, but not limited to, first-year students.*

    The Council recommends that Congress give serious consideration to the establishment of a National Student Loan Bank to replace existing student loan programs, as recommended in its report, The Federal Role in Postsecondary Education.

---

[9]This estimate is based on analysis of student borrowers in general, not on those in the health professions in particular. With their relatively high incomes, physicians and dentists might have a shorter average repayment period, but, on the other hand, they tend to borrow larger amounts before completing their education than the average student.

6

New Medical and Dental Schools?

The rapid increase in the size of entering medical school classes that has occurred since the late 1960s suggests a need for great caution in supporting the establishment of any more new medical schools, especially in view of the exceedingly large expenditures needed to establish such schools. There is, however, a case for adequate geographic distribution of medical schools, in view of the evidence that a medical school tends to attract health manpower to an area. On the other hand, we are beginning to accumulate evidence that area health education centers are also effective in attracting health manpower to the areas in which they are located.

How Many New Medical Schools?

The Carnegie Commission expressed the view that there should be a university health science center in every metropolitan area with a population of 350,000 or more, except for those areas that could benefit from centers existing in other geographically convenient communities. After eliminating a number of communities that were located relatively close to existing medical schools, the Commission identified nine areas in which new medical schools should be established. In the period since 1970, medical schools, or clinical branches of existing medical schools, have been established in seven of these areas and an area health education center in an eighth (Table 2). However, new medical

Table 2. Communities for which Carnegie Commission (1970) recommended
new medical schools, and medical schools or other facilities developed
in those communities since 1970

Community	Population, 1972 (000)	Name and status of school or other facility	Control	Veterans Administration funding
Phoenix, Arizona	1,053	Clinical training center	Public	
Fresno, California	431	Area health education center	Public	x
Wilmington, Delaware	512			
Jacksonville, Florida	636	Clinical training center	Public	
Wichita, Kansas	376	Clinical branch of University of Kansas School of Medicine	Public	
Springfield, Massachusetts	591	Clinical training center	Mixed	
Duluth, Minnesota	267	University of Minnesota, Duluth, developing, operational	Public	
Tulsa, Oklahoma	560	College of Osteopathic Medicine and Surgery	Public	
		Clinical branch of University of Oklahoma School of Medicine	Public	
Norfolk, Virginia	729	Eastern Virginia Medical School, developing, operational	Private[a]	

[a]The school is classified as private in publications of the Council on Medical Education, American Medical Association, but it considers itself "community-based," with substantial support from various community agencies, as well as from the State of Virginia.

Source: Developed from various sources, including "Medical Education in the United States, 1974-75" (1975).

schools are being developed in 13 communities in which the Commission did not recommend a new school (Table 3). These 13 schools have all reached the planning stage in which a dean has been appointed, but have not yet enrolled students. A number of other communities have also been attempting to promote plans for new medical schools.

An important factor in the establishment of five of the schools included in Table 3 was the enactment of the Veterans

Table 3. New medical schools developing in communities other than
those recommended by Carnegie Commission (1970)

Location	Population, 1972 (000)	Name and status of school	Control	Veterans Administration funding
Window Rock, Arizona	1 (1970)	Navajo Medical School	Public	
Atlanta, Georgia	1,684	Morehouse College Medical Education Program	Private	
Macon, Georgia	232	Mercer University School of Medicine, developing	Private	
Rochester, Minnesota	87	Mayo Medical School, developing, operational	Private	
Greenville, North Carolina	29 (1970)	East Carolina University School of Medicine	Public	
Dayton, Ohio	857	Wright State University School of Medicine, developing	Public	x
Kent, Ohio (Akron Metropolitan area)	676	Northeastern Ohio Universities College of Medicine, developing	Public	
Columbia, South Carolina	336	University of South Carolina Medical School, developing	Public	x
Johnson City, Tennessee	33 (1970)	East Tennessee State University	Public	x
Fort Worth, Texas	356	Texas College of Osteopathic Medicine[a]	Private	
College Station, Texas (Bryan-College Station Metropolitan area)	62	Plans for school to be conducted jointly by Baylor University and Texas A&M University	Public	x
Huntington, West Virginia	293	Marshall University School of Medicine, developing	Public	x
Bethesda, Maryland (Washington, D.C. Metropolitan area)	2,999	University of Health Sciences of the Uniformed Services[b]	Public	

[a]Not listed in "Medical Education in the United States, 1974-75."

[b]Authorized by the Uniformed Services Health Professions Revitalization Act of 1972 (Public Law 92-426).

Sources: Compiled from various sources, including "Medical Education in the United States, 1974-75" (1975).

Administration Medical School Assistance and Health Manpower Training Act of 1972 (Public Law 92-541), which authorized (1) a program of VA assistance to states for the establishment of new medical schools, (2) a program of grants to medical schools that have maintained affiliations with the VA, and (3) a program of grants to affiliated institutions to assist in the coordination, improvement, and expansion of allied health education. In 1973-74, five institutions applied to the VA for financial assistance in starting new medical schools. All five, after meeting certain conditions, received VA approval of grant applications, with a combined potential initial award of nearly $17,000,000. They are the five institutions designated as having VA funding in Table 3.[1]

We are not suggesting that all of the schools listed in Table 3 are excessive. In fact, we believe that special consideration should be given to medical education programs that are particularly likely to encourage members of minority groups to train for the medical profession, in view of the extremely small proportions of minority groups among physicians. Historically, Howard University College of Medicine and Meharry Medical College have been the only medical schools enrolling significant numbers of black students and have played important roles in the training of black physicians. With Howard located in Washington, D.C., and Meharry in Nashville, Atlanta would be a logical third place for a medical education program designed to encourage the training of black physicians, and we believe that the several affiliated institutions combined in the Atlanta University Center provide a potential base for such a program. The developing program in Window Rock, Arizona, which is designed for the training of Navajos and is associated with an area health education center program affiliated with the University of New Mexico School of Medicine, also merits special consideration as a way of attracting Native Americans, who have scarcely been represented at all in the medical profession, to

---

[1] According to AAMC testimony before the Subcommittee on Health, U.S. Senate, eight additional schools are in development with the support of VA funds (Bennett and Cooper, 1976, p. 2056). This may include schools that had not as yet been included in AMA listings.

undertake medical training. However, we are doubtful that either of these programs should become four-year medical schools in the foreseeable future.

With respect to most of the developing schools listed in Table 3, we seriously question whether they should be established.[2] We also question whether the VA should have been given authority to provide funds for new medical schools independently of the Health Resources Administration in the U.S. Public Health Service, the agency within the federal government responsible for administering most of the aid to university health science centers. It is also interesting to note that in both South Carolina and Tennessee, state legislatures approved the establishment of the new schools (in Columbia, South Carolina, and Johnson City, Tennesee) in the face of opposition (at least initially) by those states' respective commissions on higher education, which favored instead the development of a network of area health education centers. There is reason to believe that the possibility of VA funds was a major factor in those decisions.

Existing and developing university health science centers and recommended new centers are shown in Map 1, along with developing schools that are not recommended by the Carnegie Council. A number of the new public medical schools that we consider excessive have been approved by the appropriate state agencies—in some cases after considerable controversy.

A number of interrelated considerations are involved in our warning that we are developing too many new medical schools: (1) the increase in medical-school entrants and graduates was even more pronounced in the first half of the 1970s than had been predicted and will continue to be substantial for a number of years without the contributions of schools that have not yet enrolled any students; (2) it is a virtual certainty that the physician-population ratio will reach unprecedented levels by 1985, even if the net inflow of FMGs is drastically curtailed; (3) the cost of establishing a new medical school is exceedingly high; and (4) communities that lack a medical school

---

[2]For a similar warning, see Carnegie Foundation for the Advancement of Teaching (1976).

Map 1. University health science centers and schools of osteopathy, developing centers, and Carnegie Council recommendations for new health centers

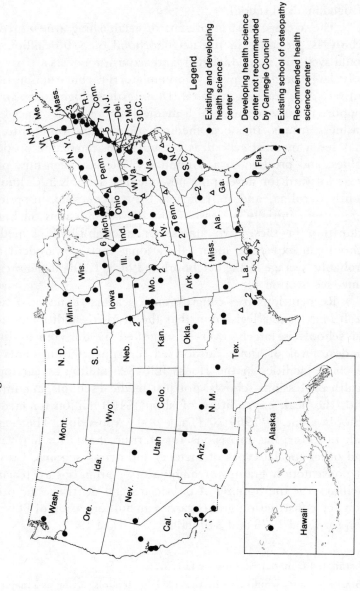

Legend

● Existing and developing health science center

△ Developing health science center not recommended by Carnegie Council

■ Existing school of osteopathy

▲ Recommended health science center

Sources: "Medical Education in the United States, 1974-75" (1975); and other sources.

can, in most cases, be served more effectively and at much more modest cost by an area health education center than by a full-fledged medical school.

The average cost at present of establishing a new medical school is probably in the neighborhood of $100 million.[3] It could well run much higher if land acquisition costs are particularly large or if the plans contemplate the construction of an entirely new teaching hospital. Despite these high costs, strong support for development of a medical school often comes from business groups, the local medical society, and other interests that see a medical school as bringing jobs, increased property values, and prestige to a community. We have seen how plans went forward for developing new medical schools in Columbia, South Carolina, and in Johnson City, Tennessee, in spite of opposition, initially at least, from the commissions on higher education in these two states. Once established, a medical school can expect to incur educational costs per student that probably average in the neighborhood of $11,000 at the present time (see Section 4).

Recognition by congressional leaders concerned with health-manpower legislation that the need for additional medical schools is largely over is suggested by the comparatively modest level of funds authorized for construction grants for teaching facilities in the House bill—$25 million a year for all health professions schools, not just medical schools, in contrast with the peak expenditure of about $100 million for medical schools alone in 1969-70 (Table A-1, Appendix). The Senate bill, however, has provisions for start-up grants for innovative and other special types of medical and dental schools,[4] as well as construction grants for ambulatory-, primary-care teaching facilities for the training of physicians and dentists. The provision for construction grants carries an authorization of $80 million for fiscal 1978 and $40 million for fiscal 1979.

[3]Estimated from data in Smythe (1972).

[4]Start-up grants would also be provided for schools having as a major objective the training of individuals from disadvantaged backgrounds, and regional health professions schools.

We have already suggested (Section 4) that the training of physicians and dentists for ambulatory care and for some of the other special purposes contemplated in the start-up provisions can be encouraged in existing university health science centers and in area health education centers. The creation of new schools for these purposes is unwarranted.

Congress should discontinue the allocation of separate funds to the Veterans Administration for the establishment of medical schools and should centralize authority for final decisions on start-up grants and construction grants and loans for health-professions schools with the Secretary of HEW. The Veterans Administration hospitals play an important role in medical education through their affiliations in a large number of cases with medical schools, and will continue to do so, but we consider it most unwise administratively to have more than one federal agency involved in decisions about the allocation of funds for new medical schools.

How Many New Dental Schools?

Like medical schools, dental schools should have adequate geographical distribution even though new dental schools may not be needed at present purely for the purpose of accelerating the increase in dental-school enrollment. How adequate is the geographical distribution of dental schools? They are located in 32 states, as well as in the District of Columbia and Puerto Rico (Map 2). Most of the states that lack dental schools are comparatively small and/or sparsely populated. The chief exception is Arizona, with a population of nearly 2.2 million in 1974 and the highest rate of net in-migration in the early 1970s of any of the states. Moreover, there is no dental school in the neighboring states of New Mexico, Utah, and Nevada. We believe that plans for a dental school in Arizona should be developed. Florida will probably eventually need a second dental school, in addition to the one recently developed at the University of Florida. The other states that lack a dental school would in most cases be well advised to meet the needs of their residents seeking dental education by joining in regional plans under which students can attend dental schools in neighboring states

Map 2. Existing dental schools and Carnegie Council recommendations for new dental schools

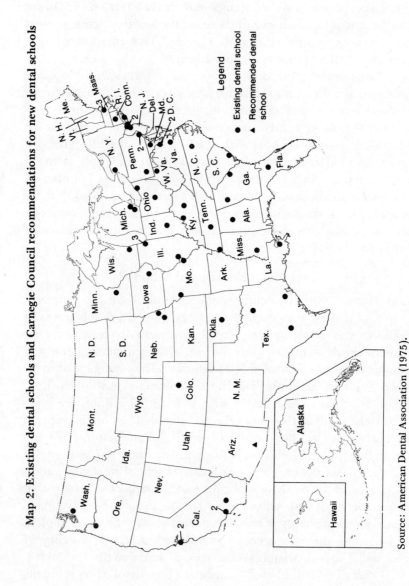

Legend

● Existing dental school

▲ Recommended dental school

Source: American Dental Association (1975).

at the tuition charge for residents of those states, with the state in which the student resides reimbursing the school for the difference between resident and nonresident tuition. A number of states participate in such plans through the New England Board of Higher Education, the Southern Regional Education Board, and the Western Interstate Commission for Higher Education.

We would urge any new dental school to be associated with a university health science center. Dental education should not take place in isolation from education in other health professions. Thus, as Map 2 suggests, the preferred location of a new dental school in Arizona would be Tucson, the location of the University of Arizona College of Medicine.

Detailed recommendation 11: *On grounds of adequate geographic distribution, the Council recommends the development of a new medical school in Wilmington, Delaware. Authority for the Veterans Administration to provide funds for new medical schools should be repealed by Congress, and all decisions relating to start-up funds and construction funds from federal sources should be centralized with the Secretary of HEW.*

Among developing medical education programs, the Council believes that special consideration should be given to programs in Atlanta, Georgia, and Window Rock, Arizona, that are designed to encourage members of minority groups to train for the medical profession.

The Council recommends the development of a new dental school in Arizona, preferably in Tucson. Apart from Arizona, states that lack a dental school should seek arrangements with neighboring states under the auspices of regional higher education boards to provide dental education for their residents, if they are not already involved in such arrangements.

Congress should authorize the Secretary of HEW to make a determination, after consultation with appropriate advisory bodies, to withhold federal funds, including capitation payments, from developing medical and dental schools deemed to be excessive.

7

Area Health
Education Centers

The formation of area health education centers has been one of the most encouraging and impressive developments under the 1971 legislation. As recommended by the Carnegie Commission, an area health education center would perform all of the functions of a university health science center except for the basic education of M.D. and D.D.S. candidates (and of students in certain other health-professions schools, such as schools of veterinary medicine and pharmacy). Centers would be located in both the ghetto areas of large cities and in communities located at some distance from a university health science center—the communities to be chosen to provide a well-distributed geographic network of centers. Each center would be affiliated with a university health science center, which would supervise its educational programs.

Their Functions

The functions of area health education centers would be as follows:

1. To maintain a community hospital of outstanding quality, many of whose patients would be admitted on a referral basis from small communities in the surrounding area.
2. To conduct educational programs under the supervision of

the faculty of the university health science center with which the area center is affiliated.
3. To have these educational programs include
   a. Residency programs;
   b. Clinical instruction for M.D. candidates and D.D.S. candidates who would come there from the university health science center on a rotating basis;
   c. Clinical experience for students in allied health programs;
   d. Continuing education programs for health manpower in the area, conducted in cooperation with local professional associations.
4. To provide guidance to comprehensive colleges and community colleges in the area in the development of training programs for allied health professions.
5. To cooperate with hospitals and community agencies in the planning and development of more effective health-care delivery systems.
6. To conduct limited research programs concerned primarily with the evaluation of health-care delivery systems.[1]

The primary purpose of area health education centers is to improve the quality of health care in their areas. But they can also play a significant role in the effort to overcome geographic maldistribution of health manpower. The majority of medical residents remain to practice in the states in which they served their residencies. In fact, several studies indicated "that a larger portion of individuals with residency training were practicing in the state of their residency than were practicing in the state of prior residence, state of medical college, or state of internship" (Fein and Weber, 1971, p. 156).[2]

[1]This definition of area health education centers, included in Carnegie Commission (1970), was adopted with scarcely any changes by the federal Bureau of Health Resources Development (U.S. Department of Health, Education, and Welfare, 1973).

[2]In interpreting this finding, it must be recognized that many M.D.s probably choose their residencies in states in which they would like to practice permanently, and indeed "the attractiveness of a state as a place to practice significantly affects the ability of hospitals in that state to attract"

Unfortunately, practically all the research has been concerned with interstate differences in the supply of physicians and does not shed much light on whether serving a residency in a particular community will strongly influence an individual's decision to practice in that community. The experience with area health education centers is too recent to yield hard statistical data on this point, but there is a good deal of anecdotal evidence indicating that development of a high-quality residency program in a community hospital has been of substantial assistance in attracting physicians to communities suffering from shortages.

The development of area health education centers received strong administration endorsement in the spring of 1971 and, as we have seen, was a main objective of the provision for "health manpower initiative awards" in the 1971 health manpower legislation. In 1972, the Bureau of Health Manpower Education entered into contracts with 11 medical schools or their parent universities in as many states to develop area health education centers.[3] Total first-year funding for these contracts was $11 million, with a five-year commitment of $65 million.[4] In addition, eight AHECs were developed under the auspices of the Veterans Administration and with substantial VA funding in 1971-72. By far the largest number of AHECs (about 100), however, have been developed under the Regional Medical

residents who are U.S. medical graduates (ibid., pp. 176-177). A more recent study by Yett and Sloan (1974) indicates that the extent of previous attachment to a state (as measured by how many of the "events" of birth, medical school education, internship, and residency occurred in a given state) had a very important influence on decisions of newly trained physicians to practice in a given state, but that the most recent of these events were more important than the more remote events. The highest probabilities of practicing in a state were associated with those combinations of events that included internships and residencies. Significantly, Yett and Sloan conclude that state investment in medical schools may be more fruitful, in terms of increasing the supply of physicians in a state, than previous studies had indicated.

[3]The functions of the Bureau of Health Manpower Education were later transferred to the Bureau of Health Resources Development.

[4]For a more detailed account of these developments, see Miike and Ross (1975).

Programs (RMP), sometimes with additional funding from other sources. The RMP centers are not usually affiliated with a university health science center and do not typically have clinical-training programs, but tend to be concerned, rather, with continuing education programs and educational development activities, such as consumer education and regional health planning.[5]

In Table A-6, Appendix, we have assembled all the available data about university health science centers, area health education centers, and other clinical or basic science training centers that are not called AHECs. Most of the information about AHECs is based on a report prepared for the Bureau of Health Resources Development by C. E. Pagan Associates, Inc. (1975), but we have added information drawn from other sources where appropriate. The Pagan Associates report used two basic classifications of AHECs:

1. *Carnegie Model Consortium*—a consortium of health-care providers and educational institutions with linkage to a central medical or university health science center that provides central coordination and is responsible for developing cooperative educational programs with and among institutions at local levels.
2. *Community-Based Consortium*—a health-manpower education consortium of local health-care providers and educational institutions which is responsible for coordinating and developing cooperative educational programs at the local level. Such a consortium may include universities, colleges, or medical schools within the local area but no single institution has central responsibility for program direction.

The basic distinction, then, between a Carnegie Model Consortium and a Community-Based Consortium is the nature

[5] A 1971 RMP discussion draft described an AHEC as concerned with the "connection between the health service needs defined by community health planning agencies and the manpower recruitment and education resources . . . . The concept of an AHEC as a satellite of the University Health Science Center implies a relationship which RMPs does not endorse" (quoted in ibid., pp. 246-247).

of the relationship or lack of it with a university health science center. Beyond that, the report subclassifies AHECs according to their functions. Those with comprehensive programs have clinical, continuing, and educational development activities. Those that are not classified as comprehensive have only one or two of these three types of activities. Clinical education activities include any training program that leads to the attainment of a degree, certificate, or license in a health profession. Continuing education activities include any training program provided for health professionals to expand their skills but not usually leading to a certificate or degree. Educational development activities cover a broad range, including public or consumer education, counseling, recruitment and retention activities, planning or evaluation, and other similar functions.

The community-based consortia tend to have received their funding from RMPs although there are sometimes combinations of sources of funds. While performing highly useful functions, they cannot be considered fully developed AHECs, because the central core of an AHEC program, as conceived by the Carnegie Commission and as endorsed by the Bureau of Health Resources Development, is the development of clinical-training programs, especially for physicians and dentists and for physician's and dentist's assistants, in community hospitals under the supervision of a university health science center with which the AHEC is affiliated. It is this activity of an AHEC, above all, that can be expected to improve the quality of health care and help to overcome shortages of health manpower in an area. We would add that clinical training, especially in dentistry, may take the form of a preceptorship rather than hospital-based training, but it should be conducted under the supervision of the faculty of a university health science center and closely tied to an AHEC.

Because we regard clinical training programs as the central core of a fully developed AHEC program, we consider affiliation with a university health science center essential. There can be little dispute over the need for health science center supervision over clinical training in an AHEC setting for M.D. and D.D.S. candidates, and the clear preferences of U.S. medical graduates for residency programs affiliated with a medical school are just one of the many types of evidence that close supervision by faculty members of a university health science center is considered indispensable for a high-quality residency program.

In Map 3, we have identified those AHECs that are affiliated with university health science centers and have clinical-training activities. Some of them are more appropriately characterized as area health education systems, embracing activities over a number of counties, rather than as centers. In those cases, we have shaded in a portion of a state to indicate the area covered.[6]

Although the development of area health education centers received decided impetus from the Carnegie Commission recommendation and the federal administrative and legislative developments of 1971, it is important to recognize that a number of antecedents involving elements of the concept of an area health education center or system, if not called by these names, had existed for some time. Several individual hospitals, notably the Mary I. Bassett Hospital in Cooperstown, New York, had carefully supervised residency programs. The renowned Mayo Clinic, with its worldwide reputation, also had a less-noticed impact on the quality of medical care in southeastern Minnesota.[7] The Duke Foundation had been financing a program to improve the quality of care in rural North Carolina and South Carolina for 35 to 40 years and Bingham Associates, centered in

[6]The concept of area health education systems, as opposed to single centers, was urged by Swanson (1972, p. 325). "Rather than recreating uncoordinated, semi-autonomous" centers, "it is proposed that Area Health Education and Delivery Systems (AHEADS) be developed." In fact, to the extent that a number of AHECs would be linked with a single coordinating university health science center (or with several cooperating health science centers) under the Carnegie Commission proposal, a system comparable to that envisaged by Swanson would emerge. This is precisely what has happened in several states, notably North Carolina and South Carolina.

[7]Patients with complex medical problems are referred to the Mayo Clinic from all parts of the United States and also from foreign countries, but a physician located in southeastern Minnesota would be especially likely to refer a patient or to seek advice from the Mayo staff.

Map 3. Existing area health education centers, area health education systems, and other decentralized clinical training facilities

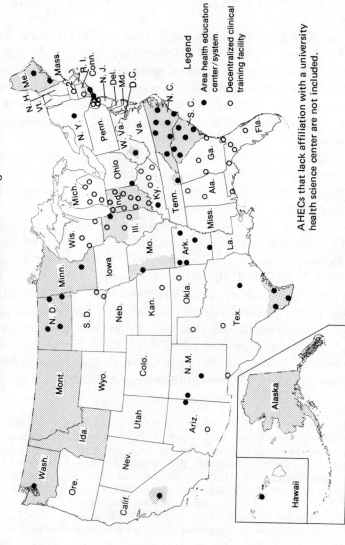

Legend

● Area health education center/system

○ Decentralized clinical training facility

AHECs that lack affiliation with a university health science center are not included.

Source: Table A-6, Appendix.

Boston, conducted programs to improve the quality of hospital care throughout the State of Maine.

Sometimes neglected in discussions of AHECs, however, have been the efforts of individual states in recent years to encourage decentralized medical education training programs, family-practice residency programs, and other related programs —usually with central involvement of a public medical school or group of medical schools. By 1974, nine states had significant developments of this type, and three others had them under serious consideration ("State Funding for Targeted Programs . . . ," 1974).

Probably the pioneering effort along these lines was in the State of Indiana, which established the Indiana Statewide Medical Education System in 1967 to increase and redistribute physician manpower in the state. By 1974, clinical training for M.D. candidates at Indiana University School of Medicine was provided in 50 affiliated community hospitals throughout the state and graduate residency training in seven communities. In the first four years, state funds amounting to $5.5 million were expended to pay stipends for interns and residents, support salaries of community hospital directors of medical education, and pay expenses of visiting professors. Later, as Table A-6, Appendix, indicates, funds were obtained from the U.S. Department of Health, Education, and Welfare to support the program.[8] By 1974, 55 percent of graduates of the medical school were staying on to pursue their residency training in the state, apparently a decided improvement over the earlier experience.[9]

North Carolina represents a particularly interesting exam-

---

[8] The Pagan Associates report (1975) indicates that state funds supported the program until 1971 and HEW funds thereafter, but we have included state funds as a source in 1972-75 in the table, because they were so important in the development of the program.

[9] See Lee (1975, p. 383) for a discussion of these results. Lee also mentions Wisconsin as having a similar program, but the Wisconsin program is considerably more limited, involving some clinical training for medical-school juniors in La Crosse, Marshfield, and Milwaukee, and a certain number of preceptorships for seniors (information provided by the dean's office, University of Wisconsin Medical School).

ple of a state that (through the University of North Carolina School of Medicine) was awarded one of the BHRD contracts for development of AHECs but has also allocated substantial state funds for its AHEC program. In fact, the school of medicine began to enter into affiliation arrangements with various community hospitals in 1967, and at about the same time the other health science schools on the Chapel Hill campus—dentistry, nursing, pharmacy, and public health began "community outreach" programs (U.S. Department of Health, Education, and Welfare, 1973, p. 15). In 1969, the state legislature began to provide funds for the development of graduate and undergraduate medical education programs in the affiliated hospitals. The next step was the BHRD five-year contract, providing $8.5 million for the development of three AHECs. In 1974, the legislature appropriated $28.5 million to develop six additional AHECs and to augment the existing ones.

The nine AHECs provide North Carolina with a comprehensive network of regional centers designed to meet the health-manpower development needs of all 100 counties in the state. From the state funds, $23.5 million are being used for the construction of appropriate educational facilities at each of the nine AHECs, which are centered around existing community hospitals. Some of the centers have several community hospitals as their nucleus, and each of the nuclear community hospitals develops relationships with hospitals in smaller communities to upgrade the quality of health care they provide and to improve their access to sophisticated equipment.

There are now three university medical centers—Duke, UNC, and Bowman Gray—involved in the effort. By the spring of 1975, 40 full-time medical faculty members were based in the AHECs, along with 20 full-time faculty in other health disciplines. Plans involved increasing these numbers to 80 and 50, respectively, by 1980. The teaching faculties of the centers also include substantial numbers of local practitioners who teach on a part-time basis.

Other highlights of the North Carolina program include:

1. Gradually increasing the proportion of clinical education of
   M.D. candidates given off campus to about one-third by

1980; development of 300 new primary-care residency positions, of which 200 will be in family practice, by 1980; and provision of residency training in primary care in community hospitals

2. Four weeks spent in an AHEC setting by each senior in the UNC dental school

3. One-half of a semester spent in an AHEC setting by each senior in the school of pharmacy

4. Time spent in AHEC settings by many of the students in the school of public health

5. Rotation of both undergraduate and graduate students at the UNC school of nursing through periods at the AHECs; development of cooperative relationships with other nurse-training programs in the state to assure a network of high-quality educational programs that serve regional needs

6. Continuing education for health manpower, and a program of regular visits by UNC medical faculty to a number of communities across the state to see patients referred by local physicians.[10]

Each of the BHRD AHEC programs has its own distinctive characteristics, but all give emphasis to decentralized health-manpower training, in many cases with particular reference to M.D. candidates and physician residency training. As we have suggested in Section 3, AHECs are especially suitable for the development of primary-care residency programs, which can be conducted effectively in community hospitals, whereas university teaching hospitals have advantages for more specialized training, because they tend to admit complex and difficult cases on a referral basis. AHEC programs are also well adapted to the training of physician's assistants, nurse practitioners, and dental auxiliary personnel. One of the more interesting of the AHEC programs is that of the University of North Dakota, which has placed special emphasis on physician preceptorships and on the

---

[10]This discussion of the North Carolina program is based on U.S. Department of Health, Education, and Welfare (1973, pp. 15-17) and papers included in U.S. Department of Health, Education, and Welfare (1976a).

training of pediatric nurse assistants, family-practice nurse practitioners, and nurse midwives.

A very recent addition to the roster of states that are putting state funds into decentralized health-manpower training is Maryland, where legislation has been enacted that will provide funds for a program under which five AHECs will be developed in appropriate communities throughout the state.[11] The program is aimed particularly at increasing the supply of primary-care physicians in underserved areas, which, it is believed, cannot be accomplished simply by increasing medical-school enrollment ("Medical Center Eyed . . . ," 1976).

The North Carolina experience and the initiative taken in a number of states toward decentralization of medical and dental clinical training strongly suggest the desirability of a more explicit federal-state partnership in the support of AHECs. We believe that a portion of federal funds for AHECs should be allocated to states that are prepared to come up with matching funds and that are developing state plans for AHECs.

Their Location

The geographic distribution of fully developed AHECs represents, on the one hand, very encouraging progress in a relatively short period of time and, on the other, obviously quite spotty and uneven coverage (Map 3). Thirty-three states have AHECs or clinical training centers or area health education systems under the supervision of a university health science center. Only in about four of these states is there comprehensive coverage of all parts of the state. And some of the programs are of very limited scope—for example, the decentralized clinical training centers in Wisconsin.

All in all, there are about 55 area health education centers or clinical training centers and about 13 area health education systems that cover substantial numbers of counties, entire states, or even groups of states, as in the Washington-Alaska-Idaho-Montana system affiliated with the University of Wash-

[11]Information provided by the Dean's Office, University of Maryland School of Medicine.

ington School of Medicine. Clearly there is enormous variation in the activities of these centers. Where area health education systems cover very large areas, as in the four-state group centered around the University of Washington School of Medicine, it may be assumed that development of full-fledged area centers is somewhat spotty and in an early stage. Even so, the organizational structure may be assumed to be in place, and we have not suggested specific additional area health education centers for such areas, nor for those communities that have very limited clinical-training centers. With continued financial support from federal and state governments and from private sources, many of these systems and centers can develop into fully developed AHECs.[12]

We have listed about 70 additional suggested centers in Table A-6, Appendix. Where we have indicated a suggestion for a "fully developed center," a center that is not affiliated with a university health science center already exists, most often having been supported by RMP funds. The majority of these centers have continuing education programs and/or educational development programs. With adequate financial support, they could become full-fledged AHECs. Meanwhile, we do not by any means intend to downgrade their activities in continuing education and health education, to which we attach great importance.

Thus far, most of our discussion has been concerned with the activities of medical schools in developing decentralized training. There has also been a substantial movement in recent years to provide some of the dental student's clinical training in sites removed from the dental school. In 1975, it was reported that 29 dental schools had training of this type, and the settings in which it was provided were quite varied. They included mobile clinics, field experiences with migrant farmers, private offices in underserved urban and/or rural areas, nursing- and old-age-home experiences, centers for treating exceptional chil-

[12]We cannot be certain that Table A-6, Appendix, and Map 3 include every clinical training center associated with a university health science center although we have made every effort to develop a comprehensive list.

dren, prisons, hospital clinics in underserved areas, and satellite clinics treating drug addicts (Redig, 1975, p. 608). In the fall of 1975, the AADS published the results of a special survey that indicated that 52 dental schools (out of 54 responding schools) had off-campus training (American Association of Dental Schools, 1975b). The most common sites for such training were hospitals and public clinics, and, interestingly, 44 of the responding schools reported off-campus facilities in inner-city areas, while 29 indicated they had training programs in rural areas. Some of the decentralized dental training, of course, is associated with AHECs, as we saw in the North Carolina case.

The University of Washington School of Dentistry is developing a plan under which students from such states as Idaho and Montana (which have no dental schools) will be enrolled in the dental school of the University of Washington but will have at least some of both their preclinical and clinical education in their home states. The University of Washington School of Medicine has had a similar program for some time.

The legislation now before Congress would provide additional funds for AHECs, and both the Senate and House Bills include provisions that call for affiliation of AHECs with university health science centers and that in other ways conform to the criteria listed at the beginning of this section. We believe, as suggested above, that some of the funds allocated for AHECs should take the form of matching funds for states that develop plans for AHECs. Many of the existing centers that were started under the RMP program could provide the nucleus for fully developed AHECs in a number of states.

Thus far, development of AHECs in inner-city areas has not been given a great deal of emphasis, although there are some examples of such programs, including the Metro Six Hospital group in Chicago, which is part of the Illinois Area Health Education System under the supervision of the University of Illinois College of Medicine. A few similar programs also originated under the former U.S. Office of Economic Opportunity, like the Martin Luther King Center in the Bronx (New York City), which is affiliated with the Albert Einstein School of Medicine. However, so far as we have been able to determine, only a few of the OEO centers had clinical-training programs for physicians or dentists, and very few of them had any formal ties with AHECs.[13]

The Carnegie Commission (1970) suggestions for the location of AHECs did not specifically include many large cities, because it was assumed that decentralized health education programs would develop under the auspices of the university health science centers that exist in large cities. This has happened in certain instances but not as yet very extensively.

Whether or not AHECs have developed in particular states and communities has thus far depended on the initiative of certain university health science centers in seeking federal funds for the purpose, action taken at the state level, or VA initiative in some cases. In the future administration of federal funds for the development of AHECs, there should be special emphasis on seeking out appropriate sponsors in states and areas that as yet have little or no involvement. Map 4 indicates communities for which we suggest additional fully developed AHECs.[14]

Our suggestions for about 70 additional AHECs would bring the total number of AHECs and clinical-training centers, including those that are parts of systems, above the 126 centers suggested by the Carnegie Commission in 1970. The reason for this is that some of the clinical-training centers, for example, in Kentucky, are in very small communities and thus do not meet the needs of larger communities. As in the Commission's 1970

[13]For information on OEO centers, which are now under the auspices of the Bureau of Community Health Services of HEW, see Hollister, Kramer, and Bellin (1974) and U.S. Department of Health, Education, and Welfare (1975b).

[14]The North Carolina experience, in particular, suggests that the 1970 proposal of the Carnegie Commission for 126 AHECs was quite modest. For a state with three established medical schools and one developing school, the Commission suggested three AHECs in communities relatively remote from those schools. Assuming that two AHECs would develop within the areas of existing medical schools (Duke and UNC are so close together that they are within the same area), the Commission was essentially identifying a need for five AHECs. The state, as we have seen, has developed nine, and that number by no means seems excessive. Actually, the Commission deliberately held down the number of suggested centers to avoid appearing to propose an unreachable goal.

Map 4. Carnegie Council suggestions for additional area health education centers

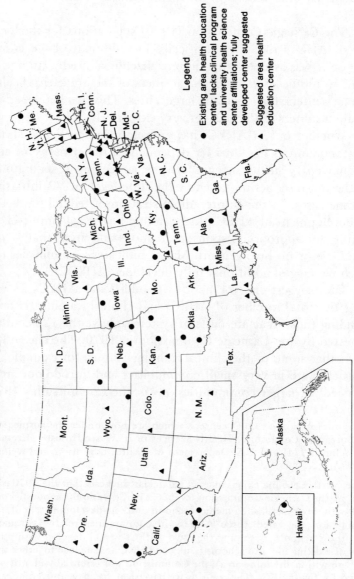

Legend

● Existing area health education center, lacks clinical program and university health science center affiliations; fully developed center suggested

▲ Suggested area health education center

[a]Under recently enacted state legislation, five AHECs are to be developed in Maryland.

report, locations of centers are being suggested, but not firmly recommended. Final choices of locations should be made on the basis of careful regional and local planning that takes account, among other things, of the relative quality of community hospitals in various communities. Our suggestions are made, as were those in the 1970 report, with a view to giving a general idea of how many additional centers are needed.

Another point that should be kept in mind is that some of the developing medical schools that are "not recommended" by the Council are in communities where an AHEC should be developed.

We do not believe that every university health science center should necessarily become equally involved in developing clinical training at centers remote from its central teaching facilities. In fact, some of the leading schools, such as Johns Hopkins and Harvard, have not, with certain minor exceptions, developed remote clinical facilities but have become extensively involved in sponsoring prepaid health-care plans and other efforts in inner-city and nearby areas. Some medical schools will continue to be especially noted for their research programs, and this is as it should be. Although we believe that every university health science center should become more concerned with efforts to improve the quality of health care in its area than has been traditional, these efforts can take a variety of forms, and federal policy should not be directed toward imposing a single model on each and every school.[15] It is for this reason that we oppose provisions making capitation payments conditional on conducting a certain proportion of a school's clinical training in sites remote from its main teaching facility.

Enactment of the National Health Planning and Resources Development Act of 1975 left the future of area centers developed by Regional Medical Programs (RMPs) uncertain.[16] A major purpose of the law was to establish health service areas that would be "more manageable than the multiple and often

[15] For a discussion of these issues, see Carnegie Commission (1970, Section 6).

[16] Public Law 93-641, January 4, 1975.

overlapping geographic areas developed for the comprehensive health planning, regional medical and Hill-Burton programs" (U.S. Senate, Committee on Appropriations, 1975, p. 521). Each health service area would have, with certain exceptions, no fewer than 500,000 or more than 3,000,000 persons. In contrast, some of the RMPs covered an entire state, while some had jurisdictions extending across several states. The new legislation also contemplated the establishment, within each health service area, of a health systems agency, which might take the form of a nonprofit private corporation, a public regional planning body, or a single unit of general local government if the health service area was identical to the jurisdiction of that unit. Considerable emphasis was to be placed, not only on seeking to ensure adequate health services in the area, but also on preventing unnecessary duplication of health resources and seeking means of controlling cost increases. Actual provision of services was to take the form primarily of demonstration projects rather than of on-going health care.

The new legislation has received considerable criticism, and, as yet, little information is available on its impact. We believe, however, that many of the area centers developed under the Regional Medical Programs could form the nuclei of fully developed AHECs affiliated with a university health science center. Whether this occurs or not will depend a good deal on the policies followed by the Bureau of Health Resources Development in administering the funds that will become available under health-manpower legislative proposals and on the more explicit federal-state partnership that we suggest.[17] In addition, final authority to approve allocation of federal funds for an AHEC, as for a new university health science center, should rest only with the Secretary of HEW. While VA funds have been valuable in encouraging the development of eight AHECs, as we have seen, the VA should not make separate determinations on the location of AHECs. Similarly, final decisions about the loca-

---

[17]According to Miike and Ross (1975, p. 249), "while the RMP seems destined to cease as a specific governmental program, its more successful regional programs can be expected to survive under other auspices."

tion of any AHECs developed under the new health service agencies should be coordinated with decisions of the BHRD in administering special-project grants under health manpower legislation. The involvement of three agencies in developing AHECs has been antithetical to good planning.

Future Needs

We believe that the progress that has been made in some of the states, such as North Carolina, that have developed comprehensive AHEC networks, indicates clearly that support for more extensive development of AHECs should be an important aspect of federal policy. In the future, there should be increased emphasis on reaching areas not yet involved, including inner-city areas, and a more explicit federal-state relationship (including matching federal funds) in the development of decentralized health education programs. There should also be greater coordination of all the federal programs that are involved in the broader effort to overcome geographic maldistribution and overspecialization. In fact, some provisions of legislative proposals now before Congress, such as giving special consideration to communities that will utilize physician's assistants in approving applications for assignment of a NHSC unit (see Section 5) very much move along these lines.

Detailed recommendation 12: *The Council strongly supports the continued development of area health education centers along the lines of current legislative proposals and recommends that the Secretary of HEW be given authority to use some of the federal funds for matching grants to states that are seeking to develop AHECs.*

Final authority for approval of allocation of federal funds for the development of AHECs or area health education systems should be centralized with the Secretary of Health, Education, and Welfare.

8

State Support of Medical and Dental Education

As we indicated in Section 1, there is no clearcut relationship between a state's investment in medical education and the relative supply of physicians in the state. This is not so true of dental education, because dentists are less mobile geographically than physicians.

Nevertheless, although there continue to be wide variations among the states in their expenditures on medical and dental education, the record is one of impressive progress in many states. State expenditures on medical education increased from $253 per $1,000,000 personal income in 1965-67 to $479 in 1973-74 (Table A-7, Appendix). Data are less accessible for dental education, but the AADS reports total state expenditures of $118 million on dental education, or $102 per $1,000,000 personal income, in 1974-75 (American Dental Association, n.d.).[1]

Although many states have historically been exporters of their M.D. graduates, while others—notably California for many years—have imported physicians trained in other states, there are strong forces influencing states to support medical education. For one thing, recent research has suggested a closer rela-

[1]A very small fraction of this amount was from local governments.

tionship between a state's support of medical education than had earlier been thought (Yett and Sloan, 1974). The tendency for a large proportion of medical residents to stay on and practice in the state in which they had their residency training has long been recognized, and high-quality residency programs tend to be those that are affiliated with medical schools. In addition, there has been evidence for some years that many communities that would be more effectively served by an AHEC have been seeking to develop the financial resources to establish a medical school.

In 1973-74, state expenditures on medical education ranged from $1,647 per $1,000,000 personal income in Vermont to a very small amount in Delaware (Map 5). Not surprisingly, states with predominantly public medical schools tend to spend more on medical education than states in which a substantial percentage of enrollment is in private medical schools. In this respect, financing of medical schools parallels state financing of higher education in general.[2] The states with the lowest expenditures are those with no medical schools. Their modest expenditures subsidize medical education of their residents in neighboring states, usually under regional arrangements.

The particularly high expenditures in Vermont as a percentage of personal income are explained partly by the fact that the state's public medical school has long enrolled a substantial proportion of students from other states, especially neighboring New England states, and partly by Vermont's low total personal income. Among public medical schools, which generally give preference to state residents, Vermont has by far the lowest percentage (47 percent) of its enrollment comprised of state residents (Association of American Medical Colleges, 1976a, p. 14). Legal residents of Massachusetts, Maine, and Rhode Island are given preference after state residents, and, through the New England Board of Higher Education, students from Massachusetts and Rhode Island pay resident tuition, while those from Maine pay varying tuition rates according to financial need

[2]See Carnegie Foundation for the Advancement of Teaching (1976).

Map 5. State expenditures on educational and general-purpose programs of medical schools, per $1 million personal income, 1973-74

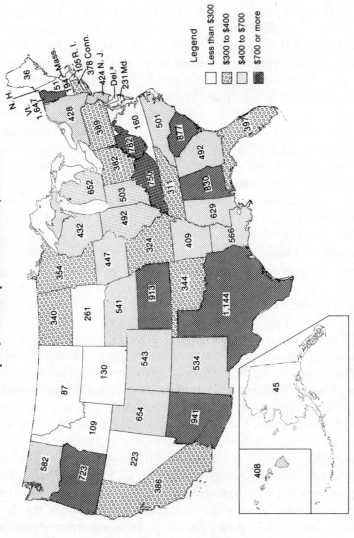

Legend

Less than $300

$300 to $400

$400 to $700

$700 or more

[a]Delaware spends a small amount on medical education; exact amount not available.

Source: "State Roles in Financing Medical Education" (1976).

(Association of American Medical Colleges, 1976a, p. 14). Although the University of Vermont College of Medicine receives subsidies for these students through the NEBHE arrangement, these subsidies plus resident tuition do not cover full costs of education.

In recent years, there have been strong pressures within states to provide support for private medical schools. These pressures were particularly intense toward the end of the 1960s when many private medical schools were experiencing severe financial problems. During this period the federal government provided a number of financial distress grants, which in many cases went to the weaker private medical schools. Even some of the strongest of the private medical schools, however, such as those at the University of Chicago and Johns Hopkins, were experiencing severe financial difficulties in the late 1960s and early 1970s, in considerable part because they were not adequately reimbursed for indigent patients served by their teaching hospitals.[3] State-supported medical schools have received subsidies in many of the states for their care of such patients.

It became clear in many states that provision of capitation payments for private medical schools that were experiencing financial difficulties would be far more economical than financing the expansion of public medical school capacity that might be needed if the private schools were forced to close their doors. Whereas Fein and Weber (1971) indicated that five states were providing financial support for private medical schools and four others were seriously considering such support, the most recent available data, for 1974-75 indicate that 33 states were providing some support for private medical schools (Table A-8, Appendix).[4] Of the 17 states that were not providing such support, 14 had no private medical school. This left only three states—Connecticut, Missouri, and Nebraska—that had one or more private medical schools and no program of support.

Among the 33 states that provide some support to private

[3]See the discussion in Carnegie Commission (1972, pp. 136-139).

[4]However, Fein and Weber's data did not cover regional arrangements, which were already in existence at that time.

medical education, however, the extent of support varies enormously. The largest programs of support are in those states, such as Florida, New York, Ohio, Pennsylvania, and Texas, that provide capitation payments to their private medical schools—in some cases limited to the number of state residents enrolled and in others not. Also of significant scope are the programs, such as those in California and Illinois, that provide capitation payments for additions to enrollment in private medical schools. More modest are the state programs, such as that of Massachusetts, that are limited to providing student aid to medical and other health-professions students. Also modest in terms of expenditures are the contributions of states—especially those with no medical schools—to subsidize medical education of their residents through the regional programs of the New England Board of Higher Education, the Southern Regional Education Board, and the Western Interstate Commission for Higher Education.[5]

In connection with this discussion of state support of private medical schools, it should be noted that the three private medical schools in the District of Columbia receive substantial special support from the federal government.

The number of states that provide support for private dental schools is considerably more limited, partly reflecting the absence in a good many states of private dental schools or any dental school at all. Table A-8, Appendix, indicates that 25 states provide some support for private dental education, but in 16 of these the support is limited to regional arrangements that may involve very limited expenditures or in some cases no expenditures. Most of the states that provide no support for

[5] Under the WICHE arrangement, students from Alaska, Arizona, Idaho, Montana, Nevada, and Wyoming can attend the participating out-of-state schools and pay only the instate tuition at public institutions and a reduced tuition at private schools. In Nevada, which now has a two-year school, the subsidies are paid for students transferring to another western school for their third and fourth years. The SREB regional plan is more limited, providing subsidies for reduced tuition at Meharry Medical College for certain students from Alabama, Florida, Georgia, Louisiana, Maryland, Mississippi, North Carolina, and Virginia (Association of American Medical Colleges, 1976, p. 14). However, Georgia's capitation payments for Emory University School of Medicine are paid through SREB.

private dental schools have no private school or no dental school. However, five states—California, Georgia, Missouri, Nebraska, and New Jersey—have one or more private dental schools and no program of support for those schools.

Data on state expenditures, however, suggest that support of private dental education is not very much out of line with support of private medical education. In 1974-75, dental schools received $14.9 million from state and interstate compact sources. The total included a very small amount from local sources (American Dental Association, n.d.). For medical education, the most recent data are for 1973-74, indicating a total of $44.6 million ("State Roles in Financing Medical Education," 1976). Thus private dental schools receive roughly one-third of the amount received by private medical schools from states and interstate sources, while their enrollment is about 40 percent of enrollment in private medical schools.

In Section 4, we pointed out that a good many dental schools are very small, with entering classes well below 100 in size. Some of these are private schools that would have difficulty expanding even with the help of federal subsidies unless they received some support from state sources. For this and other reasons, there is a case for state support of private dental schools in the states that have private schools but no programs of support.

In the preceding section, we discussed the decentralization of medical and dental education that has occurred in a number of states. In some of these states, such as Indiana, this occurred originally in response to initiative at the state level, rather than as a result of the availability of federal funds to support the development of AHECs. The move toward decentralization has gone hand in hand with programs to encourage the development of family-practice, or, more generally, primary-care residency programs in a number of states. By 1974, at least five states—Florida, Kentucky, North Carolina, South Carolina, and West Virginia—had programs aimed both at decentralization and expansion of primary-care residencies, while such programs were also under consideration in a number of other states ("State Funding for Targeted Programs . . . ," 1974). Interestingly, even Delaware, which has no medical school, established the Delaware Institute of Medical Education and Research in 1969, to support a family-practice residency program.

All of this suggests the desirability, as we indicated in earlier sections, of a more explicit federal-state partnership that would encourage expansion of schools that are too small for economical operation, decentralization of training, and emphasis on primary-care training. We have included recommendations for federal matching grants for these purposes in Sections 4 and 7. At the state level, the most urgently needed action is adoption of programs of support of private medical and dental schools in those few states that as yet have no such programs.

Detailed recommendation 14: *The Council recommends that the states that have no programs of financial support for private medical and dental schools take immediate steps toward adoption of such programs.*

Appendix A

Statistical Tables

Table A-1. Federal obligations to medical schools, 1949-50 to 1974-75 (in millions of dollars)

Year	Total	Undergraduate medical education				Graduate (research) training	Research conduct[b]	Construction[c]	Other programs
		Capitation grants[a]	Special project grants	Scholarships	Loans				
1949-50	$ 19.9	—	—	—	—	$ 4.0	$ 8.2	$ 7.7	N.A.
1954-55	34.1	—	—	—	—	6.0	26.9	1.2	
1959-60	165.1	—	—	—	—	41.5	106.4	17.2	
1964-65	503.9	—	—	—	$ 6.6	107.2	298.7	91.4	
1965-66	557.1	$ 6.6	—	—	9.7	126.1	335.2	79.5	
1966-67	708.8	18.8	—	$1.8	13.9	160.5	373.4	112.4	$ 28.0
1967-68	735.4	20.2	$ 5.5	3.2	14.6	167.3	376.2	104.6	43.8
1968-69	821.1	21.1	19.8	5.2	14.1	170.7	413.6	100.0	76.6
1969-70	824.9	21.2	34.9	7.2	8.4	161.8	391.8	99.6	100.0
1970-71	903.8	21.8	55.2	7.1	13.2	160.6	440.6	100.2	105.1
1971-72	1,065.7	95.5	47.5	7.1	15.7	162.6	585.3	24.2	127.8
1972-73	1,065.9	102.8	34.8	6.7	19.1	125.6	618.3	60.5	98.1
1973-74	1,297.0	110.9	67.5	6.4	18.7	162.8	813.0	27.7	90.0
1974-75	1,250.6	87.6	29.9	2.9	18.5	128.0	821.5	72.0	90.2

[a]Includes grants for start-up assistance to new medical schools, and for conversion of basic science schools to schools awarding the M.D. degree, 1972-1974; prior to 1972 data refer to basic support grants.

[b]Data for years prior to 1972 do not include contracts for research; contracts amounted to $60.1 million in 1972; $78.8 million in 1973; $117.6 million in 1974, and $114.7 million (est.) in 1975.

[c]Includes funds for construction of hospitals owned by medical schools.

Source: Data provided by Association of American Medical Colleges.

Table A-2. Federal obligations to dental schools, excluding research and graduate training, 1964-65 to 1974-75
(in millions of dollars)

Year	Total	Undergraduate dental education					Division of Dental Educational Assistance[c]
		Capitation grants[a]	Special project grants[b]	Scholarships	Loans	Construction	
1964-65	$24.4				$2.9	$22.1	$2.3
1965-66	25.0	$ 3.0			4.6	22.6	2.4
1966-67	54.5	8.4		$0.8	7.1	51.9	2.6
1967-68	46.6	8.9	$ 2.7	1.5	6.8	43.4	3.0
1968-69	54.4	9.2	8.7	2.4	6.8	51.2	3.3
1969-70	62.2	9.2	13.0	3.2	3.6	58.6	3.7
1970-71	64.2	9.1	15.8	3.0	5.5	60.5	3.7
1971-72	80.4	36.1	9.0	2.9	6.6	76.7	3.7
1972-73	67.9	37.9	5.4	2.7	7.9	63.0	4.8
1973-74	80.2	41.6	9.0	2.5	7.2	73.5	6.6
1974-75	57.8	33.0	5.4	1.3	6.9	52.2[d]	5.4

[a]Includes grants for start-up assistance to new dental schools.
[b]Includes financial distress grants.
[c]Includes TEAM (Training in Expanded Auxiliary Management Programs) and continuing education.
[d]Does not include interest subsidies.

Source: Data provided by American Association of Dental Schools.

Table A-3. Enrollment of first-year medical students in the United States,
by school, 1968-69 and 1974-75

State and institution	Enrollment		Percentage change
	1968-69	*1974-75*	
United States	9,863	14,963	51.7%
Alabama			
University of Alabama	91	127	39.6
University of South Alabama	–	64	–
Arizona			
University of Arizona	32	75	134.4
Arkansas			
University of Arkansas	110	122	10.9
California			
University of California, Davis	48	100	108.3
University of California, Irvine	64	70	9.4
University of California, Los Angeles	127	147	15.7
University of California, San Diego	47	96	104.3
University of California, San Francisco	130	149	14.6
University of Southern California	74	130	75.7
Loma Linda University	103	160	55.3
Stanford University	67	94	40.3
Colorado			
University of Colorado	105	129	22.9
Connecticut			
University of Connecticut	32	64	100.0
Yale University	91	102	12.1
District of Columbia			
Georgetown University	122	208	70.5
George Washington University	115	151	31.3
Howard University	104	137	31.7
Florida			
University of Florida	65	111	70.8
University of Miami	87	132	51.7
University of South Florida	–	65	–
Georgia			
Emory University	81	105	29.6
University of Georgia	105	180	71.4
Hawaii			
University of Hawaii	–	69	–

Table A-3

State and institution	Enrollment 1968-69	1974-75	Percentage change
Illinois			
Chicago Medical School	82	107	30.5%
Northwestern University	139	173	24.5
Loyola-Stritch School of Medicine	108	136	25.9
University of Chicago	80	106	32.5
University of Illinois	205	341	66.3
Rush University	—	90	—
Southern Illinois University	—	60	—
Indiana			
Indiana University	227	310	36.6
Iowa			
University of Iowa	131	179	36.6
Kansas			
University of Kansas	128	168	31.3
Kentucky			
University of Kentucky	82	111	35.4
University of Louisville	99	138	39.4
Louisiana			
Louisiana State University, New Orleans	145	149	2.8
Louisiana State University, Shreveport	—	42	—
Tulane University	137	151	10.2
Maryland			
Johns Hopkins University	93	122	31.2
University of Maryland	136	169	24.3
Massachusetts			
Boston University	88	140	59.1
Harvard University	134	165	23.1
Tufts University	120	152	26.7
University of Massachusetts	—	66	—
Michigan			
University of Michigan	210	249	18.6
Wayne State University	135	265	96.3
Michigan State University	26	111	326.9
Minnesota			
University of Minnesota, Minneapolis	164	253	54.3
Mayo Graduate School of Medicine	—	41	—

(continued on next page)

Table A-3 *(continued)*

State and institution	Enrollment 1968-69	Enrollment 1974-75	Percentage change
Mississippi			
University of Mississippi	86	154	79.1%
Missouri			
University of Missouri, Columbia	104	112	7.7
University of Missouri, Kansas City	–	73	–
St. Louis University	133	156	17.3
Washington University, St. Louis	95	126	32.6
Nebraska			
Creighton University	88	112	27.3
University of Nebraska	99	159	60.6
New Hampshire			
Dartmouth College	–	67	–
New Jersey			
College of Medicine and Dentistry of New Jersey—Newark	85	120	41.2
College of Medicine and Dentistry of New Jersey—Rutgers	–	108	–
New Mexico			
University of New Mexico	36	75	108.3
New York			
Albany Medical College	70	108	54.3
SUNY, Buffalo	105	136	29.5
SUNY, Downstate	201	226	12.4
SUNY, Stony Brook	–	49	–
SUNY, Upstate	106	124	17.0
Albert Einstein College of Medicine	101	183	81.2
Columbia University	135	148	9.6
Cornell University	92	103	12.0
Mount Sinai College of Medicine	36	81	125.0
New York Medical College	133	330	148.1
New York University	137	177	29.2
University of Rochester	79	97	22.8
North Carolina			
University of North Carolina	76	131	72.4
Duke University	86	120	39.5
Bowman Gray School of Medicine	62	90	45.2

Table A-3

State and institution	Enrollment		Percentage change
	1968-69	*1974-75*	
North Dakota			
University of North Dakota	—	68	— %
Ohio			
University of Cincinnati	108	200	85.2
Case Western Reserve University	100	147	47.0
Ohio State University	160	239	49.4
Medical College of Ohio	—	81	—
Oklahoma			
University of Oklahoma	110	159	44.5
Oregon			
University of Oregon	92	115	25.0
Pennsylvania			
Pennsylvania State University, Hershey	49	96	95.9
Hahneman Medical College	115	175	52.2
Jefferson Medical College	194	232	19.6
Medical College of Pennsylvania	66	93	40.9
Temple University	146	186	27.4
University of Pennsylvania	132	160	21.2
University of Pittsburgh	107	140	30.8
Puerto Rico			
University of Puerto Rico	84	118	40.5
South Carolina			
Medical University of South Carolina	92	165	79.3
South Dakota			
University of South Dakota	—	65	—
Tennessee			
University of Tennessee	210	205	−2.4
Meharry Medical College	87	120	37.9
Vanderbilt University	59	83	40.7
Texas			
University of Texas, Southwestern	104	202	94.2
University of Texas, Galveston	163	209	28.2
University of Texas, Houston	—	52	—
University of Texas, San Antonio	56	122	117.9

(continued on next page)

Table A-3 *(continued)*

State and institution	Enrollment		Percentage change
	1968-69	*1974-75*	
Texas *(continued)*			
Baylor University	85	168	97.6%
Texas Tech University School of Medicine	–	45	–
Utah			
University of Utah	66	101	53.0
Vermont			
University of Vermont	75	83	10.7
Virginia			
University of Virginia	86	133	54.7
Medical College of Virginia	128	168	31.3
Eastern Virginia Medical School	–	37	–
Washington			
University of Washington	85	136	60.0
West Virginia			
West Virginia University	68	84	23.5
Wisconsin			
University of Wisconsin	105	161	53.3
Medical College of Wisconsin	110	122	10.9
Basic Science Schools:			
Minnesota			
University of Minnesota School of Medicine, Duluth	–	36	–
Nevada			
University of Nevada	–	49	–

Sources: "Medical Education in the United States, 1968-69" (1969, pp. 1462-1463), and "Medical Education in the United States, 1974-75" (1975, pp. 1410-1411).

Table A-4. Active physicians (M.D.s), by specialty,
1963, 1970, and 1973

Specialty	1963	1970	1973
Total			
Number	261,728	311,203	324,367[a]
Percent	100.0	100.0	100.0
Primary care	54.5	44.0	48.4
General practice	28.2	18.4	14.9
Family practice	–		1.8
Internal medicine	14.9	13.5	19.0
Pediatrics	5.4	6.0	6.4
Obstetrics-gynecology	6.0	6.1	6.3
Surgical specialties	19.7	21.4	21.7
General surgery	9.7	9.6	9.5
Neurosurgery	0.7	0.8	0.9
Ophthalmology	3.0	3.2	3.2
Orthopedic surgery	2.6	3.1	3.3
Otolaryngology	2.0	1.7	1.7
Plastic surgery	0.4	0.5	0.6
Thoracic surgery	0.5	0.6	0.6
Urology	1.8	1.9	1.9
Other specialties	17.6	21.5	22.7
Anesthesiology	2.9	3.5	3.8
Pathology	2.8	3.4	3.5
Radiology	3.3	4.3	4.7
Psychiatry	6.3	7.5	7.7
Dermatology	1.2	1.3	1.3
Neurology	0.7	1.0	1.2
Physical medicine	0.4	0.5	0.5
Other and unspecified	7.2	13.1	7.2

[a]Exclusive of physicians not classified.

Sources: Josiah Macy, Jr. Foundation (1976, p. 88); and U.S. Public Health Service (1974, p. 60).

Table A-5. First-year residents, by specialty, September 1, 1960, 1970, and 1973

Specialty	1963	1970	1973
Total			
Number	11,070	14,556	18,076
Percent	100.0	100.0	100.0
Primary care	39.5	37.5	43.8
General practice	3.3	1.0	1.0
Family practice	–	0.9	4.2
Internal medicine	19.8	20.9	22.9
Pediatrics	8.1	8.8	10.1
Obstetrics-gynecology	8.3	5.9	5.6
Surgical specialties	30.3	30.5	26.7
General surgery	19.2	17.3	14.9
Neurosurgery	0.9	1.0	0.8
Ophthalmology	2.6	3.2	2.7
Orthopedic surgery	3.2	3.6	3.3
Otolaryngology	1.4	1.6	1.5
Plastic surgery	0.4	0.8	1.0
Thoracic surgery	0.8	0.9	0.7
Urology	1.8	2.1	1.8
Other specialties	30.2	32.0	29.5
Anesthesiology	5.0	4.7	4.4
Child psychiatry	0.3	1.2	1.6
Neurology	1.4	1.9	2.0
Psychiatry	9.9	9.5	8.1
Pathology	6.8	5.1	5.3
Physical medicine and rehabilitation	0.5	0.7	0.8
Radiology	4.9	6.5	6.1
Miscellaneous	1.4	2.4	1.2

Sources: U.S. Public Health Service (1974, p. 64); and Josiah Macy, Jr. Foundation (1976, p. 95).

Table A-6. University health science centers, clinical training centers, and area health education centers, compared with Carnegie Commission 1970 recommendations and suggestions, by state

State and city	Institution	Type of center	Health science center affiliation	Source and amount of funding, 1972-75
ALABAMA				
Health science centers				
Birmingham (785,000)*	Medical College of Alabama			
Mobile (396,400)*	University of South Alabama (developing school, operational)			
Clinical training centers				
Huntsville (285,200)*	School of Primary Medical Care		Medical College of Alabama	Medical College of Alabama
Tuscaloosa (122,500)*	College of Community Health Sciences		Medical College of Alabama	Medical College of Alabama
Area Centers				
none				
Carnegie Council suggested centers				
Montgomery (248,400)*	[fully developed center suggested]	Area health education center		
Dothan (36,733)	[suggestion repeated]	Area health education center		
ALASKA				
Health science centers				
none				
Area centers				
	[included in Washington, Alaska, Montana, Idaho, Program, Inc.—see Washington]	Area Health Education System	University of Washington School of Medicine	
Carnegie Council suggested centers				
none				

(continued on next page)

Table A-6 (continued)

State and city	Institution	Type of center	Health science center affiliation	Source and amount of funding, 1972-75
ARIZONA				
Health science centers				
Tucson (433,500)*	University of Arizona			
Health science centers in developing stage				
Window-Rock (900)	Window-Rock Navajo Indian School	Health science center		
Clinical training centers				
Phoenix (1,172,000)*			University of Arizona College of Medicine	University of Arizona College of Medicine
Area centers				
Window Rock (900)	University of New Mexico Area Health Education Center	Comprehensive	University of New Mexico School of Medicine	
Carnegie Council suggested centers				
Flagstaff (26,117)	[suggestion repeated]	Area health education center		
ARKANSAS				
Health science centers				
Little Rock (356,100)*	University of Arkansas Medical Center			
Area centers				
(Little Rock)	Area Health Education Center Program	Comprehensive	University of Arkansas Medical Center	University of Arkansas ($2,250,000)
Jonesboro (27,050)	Northeast Arkansas Area Health Education Center	Comprehensive	University of Arkansas Medical Center	

Fayetteville (144,900)*	Northwest Arkansas Area Health Education Center	Comprehensive	University of Arkansas Medical Center
Fort Smith (172,700)*	Fort Smith Area Health Education Center	Comprehensive	University of Arkansas Medical Center
Pine Bluff (84,000)*	Pine Bluff Area Health Education Center	Comprehensive	University of Arkansas Medical Center
El Dorado (25,283)	El Dorado Area Health Education Center	Comprehensive	University of Arkansas Medical Center

CALIFORNIA

Health science centers

Davis (882,600)*	University of California		
San Francisco (3,135,900)*	University of California		
Palo Alto (1,181,600)*	Stanford University		
Loma Linda (1,213,900)*	Loma Linda University		
Los Angeles (6,926,100)*	University of California		
	University of Southern California		
Irvine (1,660,900)*	University of California		
San Diego (1,518,000)*	University of California		

Area centers

Fresno (439,400)* (serves 6 counties)	Central San Joaquin Valley Area Health Education Center	Comprehensive	University of California, Los Angeles and University of California, San Francisco	BHM ($5,205,600)

Other Carnegie Council suggested centers

Chico (19,580)	[fully developed center suggested]	Area health education center
Santa Rosa (242,600)*	[fully developed center suggested]	Area health education center
Bakersfield (337,600)*	[fully developed center suggested]	Area health education center

(continued on next page)

Table A-6 (*continued*)

State and city	Institution	Type of center	Health science center affiliation	Source and amount of funding, 1972-75
CALIFORNIA (*continued*)				
Other Carnegie Commission suggested centers (*continued*)				
Los Angeles (6,926,100)*	[3 fully developed centers suggested]	Area health education centers		
San Bernardino (1,213,900)*	[fully developed center suggested]	Area health education center		
COLORADO				
Health science centers				
Denver (1,391,100)*	University of Colorado			
Area centers				
none				
Carnegie Council suggested centers				
Grand Junction (20,170)	[suggestion repeated]	Area health education center		
Pueblo (124,300)*	[suggestion repeated]	Area health education center		
CONNECTICUT				
Health science centers				
Hartford (1,058,700)*	University of Connecticut			
New Haven (759,700)*	Yale University		Yale University School of Medicine	
Clinical training centers				
Waterbury (216,808)+				
Carnegie Council suggested centers				
Bridgeport (401,752)+	[suggestion repeated]	Area health education center		

DELAWARE

Health science centers

Recommended health science center

| Wilmington (513,300)* | [recommendation repeated] | University health science center |

Area centers

Carnegie Council suggested centers

DISTRICT OF COLUMBIA

Health science centers

Georgetown University

George Washington University

Howard University

Area centers

Carnegie Council suggested centers

FLORIDA

Health science centers

Gainesville (124,000)*	University of Florida
Tampa (1,332,900)*	University of South Florida
Miami (1,415,900)*	University of Miami

Clinical training centers

| Pensacola (263,600)* | University of Florida School of Medicine | University of Florida School of Medicine |
| Tallahassee (132,700)* | University of Florida School of Medicine | University of Florida School of Medicine |

(continued on next page)

Table A-6 *(continued)*

State and city	Institution	Type of center	Health science center affiliation	Source and amount of funding, 1972-75
FLORIDA *(continued)*				
Clinical training centers (continued)				
Mayo (793)			University of Florida School of Medicine	University of Florida School of Medicine
Lake City (10,575)			University of Florida School of Medicine	University of Florida School of Medicine
Jacksonville (674,900)*			University of Florida School of Medicine	University of Florida School of Medicine
Orlando (578,600)*			University of Florida School of Medicine	University of Florida School of Medicine
Area centers				
none				
Carnegie Council suggested centers				
none				
GEORGIA				
Health science centers				
Atlanta (1,776,000)*	Emory University			
Augusta (273,800)*	Medical College of Georgia			
Health science centers in developing stage				
Atlanta (1,776,000)*	Morehouse College Medical Education Program	First two years of medical education		
Macon (235,500)*	Mercer University (not recommended by Carnegie Council)	University health science center		
Clinical training centers				
Columbus (218,000)*			Medical College of Georgia	Medical College of Georgia
Macon (235,500)*			Medical College of Georgia	Medical College of Georgia
Savannah (199,100)*			Medical College of Georgia	Medical College of Georgia

Area centers
  none
Carnegie Council suggested centers
  none

HAWAII

Health science centers
  Honolulu (691,200)* — University of Hawaii

Area centers
  Honolulu (691,200)* — Health Manpower Education Initiative Award Program — Comprehensive — University of Hawaii School of Medicine — BHM ($600,000)

Other Carnegie Council suggested centers
  Hilo (26,353) — [fully developed center suggested]

IDAHO

Health science centers
  none

Area centers
  none — [included in Washington, Alaska, Montana, Idaho, Program, Inc.—see Washington] — Area health education system — University of Washington School of Medicine

Carnegie Council suggested centers
  none

ILLINOIS

Health science centers
  Chicago (6,971,200)* —
Chicago Medical School
Northwestern University
Loyola University of Chicago
Rush Medical College
University of Chicago
University of Illinois
Chicago College of Osteopathy

(continued on next page)

Table A-6 *(continued)*

State and city	Institution	Type of center	Health science center affiliation	Source and amount of funding, 1972-75
ILLINOIS *(continued)*				
Health science centers (continued)				
Springfield (177,500)*	Southern Illinois University			
Basic sciences and clinical training centers				
Peoria (352,000)*	Peoria School of Medicine	Basic sciences and clinical training	University of Illinois Medical Center, Chicago	University of Illinois
Rockford (364,000)*	Rockford School of Medicine	Clinical training	University of Illinois Medical Center, Chicago	University of Illinois
Urbana-Champaign (163,000)*	School of Basic Medical Sciences	Basic sciences training	University of Illinois Medical Center, Chicago	University of Illinois
Area centers and systems				
Chicago (6,971,200)* (serves 50 counties)	University of Illinois Area Health Education System	Comprehensive	University of Illinois Medical Center, Chicago	HEW ($7,020,500)
Other Carnegie Council suggested centers				
Carbondale (22,816)	[fully developed center suggested]	Area health education center		
INDIANA				
Health science centers				
Indianapolis (1,143,700)*	Indiana University			
Clinical training centers				
(Indianapolis)	Indiana System for Statewide Education	Comprehensive	Indiana University School of Medicine	State funds, HEW ($5,000,000)
Gary-Hammond (643,900)*	Indiana System for Statewide Education	Comprehensive	Indiana University School of Medicine	
South Bend (280,400)*	Indiana System for Statewide Education	Comprehensive	Indiana University School of Medicine	

Fort Wayne (373,200)*	Indiana System for Statewide Education	Comprehensive	Indiana University School of Medicine
Lafayette (112,200)*	Indiana System for Statewide Education	Comprehensive	Indiana University School of Medicine
Muncie (69,080)	Indiana System for Statewide Education	Comprehensive	Indiana University School of Medicine
Terre Haute (173,700)*	Indiana System for Statewide Education	Comprehensive	Indiana University School of Medicine
Indianapolis (1,143,700)*	Indiana System for Statewide Education	Comprehensive	Indiana University School of Medicine
Bloomington (89,100)*	Indiana System for Statewide Education	Comprehensive	Indiana University School of Medicine
Evansville (288,600)*	Indiana System for Statewide Education	Comprehensive	Indiana University School of Medicine

Area centers
none

Carnegie Council suggested centers
none

IOWA

Health science centers

Des Moines (328,400)*	College of Osteopathic Medicine and Surgery
Iowa City (46,850)	University of Iowa

Area centers
none

Carnegie Council suggested centers

Sioux City (118,500)*	[fully developed center suggested]	Area health education center
Mason City (30,491)	[fully developed center suggested]	Area health education center
Davenport (364,400)*	[suggestion repeated]	Area health education center

(continued on next page)

Table A-6 (*continued*)

State and city	Institution	Type of center	Health science center affiliation	Source and amount of funding, 1972-75
KANSAS				
Health science centers				
Kansas City (1,301,600)*	University of Kansas			
Clinical training centers				
Wichita (379,000)*	University of Kansas	Clinical branch of University of Kansas School of Medicine	University of Kansas School of Medicine	University of Kansas School of Medicine
Area centers				
none				
Carnegie Commission suggested centers				
Dodge City (14,127)	[suggestion repeated]	Area health education center		
Salina (37,714)	[fully developed center suggested]			
Topeka (179,500)*	[fully developed center suggested]			
KENTUCKY				
Health science centers				
Louisville (892,500)*	University of Louisville			
Lexington (286,300)*	University of Kentucky			
Clinical training centers				
Morehead (7,005)			University of Kentucky College of Medicine	University of Kentucky College of Medicine
Somerset (10,389)			University of Kentucky College of Medicine	University of Kentucky College of Medicine
Hindman (793)			University of Kentucky College of Medicine	University of Kentucky College of Medicine

Location (population)	Institution / status	Type of center	Affiliated medical school	Federal funding
Columbia (3,128)			University of Kentucky College of Medicine	
Cloverport (1,354)			University of Kentucky College of Medicine	
Madisonville (14,105)	Pennyrile Area Health Education System		University of Louisville School of Medicine	
Carnegie Council suggested centers				
Paducah (31,627)	[suggestion repeated]	Area health education center	University of Louisville School of Medicine	
Bowling Green (36,253)	[fully developed center suggested]			
LOUISIANA				
Health science centers				
Shreveport (343,400)*	Louisiana State University, Shreveport			
New Orleans (1,090,200)*	Louisiana State University, New Orleans			
	Tulane University			
Area centers				
none				
Carnegie Council suggested centers				
Lake Charles (149,300)*	[suggestion repeated]	Area health education center		
MAINE				
Health science centers				
none				
Area centers				
Portland/Bangor (170,081)+ (serves entire state)	Maine Medical Center, Portland, and University of Maine, Bangor	Comprehensive	Tufts University School of Medicine	BHM ($3,544,600)

(continued on next page)

Table A-6 (continued)

State and city	Institution	Type of center	Health science center affiliation	Source and amount of funding, 1972-75
MAINE (continued)				
Other Carnegie Council suggested centers				
Presque Isle (11,452)	[fully developed center suggested]			
MARYLAND[a]				
Health science centers				
Baltimore (2,140,400)*	Johns Hopkins University University of Maryland			
Health science center in developing stage				
Bethesda (3,015,390)*	Medical School of the University of Health Sciences of the Uniformed Services (not recommended by Carnegie Council)			
Area centers				
Pending under new legislation[a]				
Carnegie Council suggested centers				
Cumberland	[suggestion repeated]	Area health education center		
Hagerstown	[suggestion repeated]	Area health education center		
MASSACHUSETTS				
Health science centers				
Worcester (648,400)*	University of Massachusetts			
Boston (3,918,400)*	Boston University Harvard Medical School Tufts University			

Clinical training centers			
Springfield (589,700)*	Tufts University	Clinical training center	Tufts University School of Medicine
	University of Massachusetts	Clinical training center	University of Mass., Medical School
Area centers			
none			
Carnegie Council suggested centers			
Pittsfield (150,500)*	[suggestion repeated]	Area health education center	
MICHIGAN			
Health science centers			
East Lansing (440,600)*	Michigan State University		
Ann Arbor (250,100)*	University of Michigan		
Detroit (4,434,300)*	Wayne State University		
Pontiac (85,279)	Michigan College of Osteopathic Medicine		
Clinical training centers			
Kalamazoo (261,600)*	Michigan State University		Michigan State University
Grand Rapids (558,700)*	Michigan State University		Michigan State University
Saginaw (226,900)*	Michigan State University		Michigan State University
Lansing (440,600)*	Michigan State University		Michigan State University
Flint (522,200)*	Michigan State University		Michigan State University
Area centers			
none			
Carnegie Council suggested centers			
Detroit (4,434,300)*	[suggestion repeated]	Two area health education centers	

(continued on next page)

Table A-6 (continued)

State and city	Institution	Type of center	Health science center affiliation	Source and amount of funding, 1972-75
MINNESOTA				
Health science centers				
Duluth-Superior (262,200)*	University of Minnesota (developing school, operational)			
Minneapolis (2,010,800)*	University of Minnesota			
Rochester (88,600)*	Mayo Medical School (developing school, operational)			
Area centers				
Minneapolis (2,010,800)* (served 14 counties to June 30, 1975; after that, entire state)	University of Minnesota Area Health Education Center	Comprehensive	University of Minnesota, Minneapolis	BHM ($2,407,800)
Other Carnegie Council suggested centers				
none				
MISSISSIPPI				
Health science centers				
Jackson (278,600)*	University of Mississippi			
Area centers				
none				
Carnegie Council suggested centers				
Tupelo (20,471)	[suggestion repeated]	Area health education center		
Greenville (39,648)	[suggestion repeated]	Area health education center		
Hattiesburg (38,277)		Area health education center		

MISSOURI

Health science centers

Location	Institution	Type		Funding
Kansas City (1,301,600)*	University of Missouri, Kansas City			
	Kansas City College of Osteopathy and Surgery			
Kirksville (15,560)	Kirksville College of Osteopathy and Surgery			
Columbia (86,400)*	University of Missouri			
St. Louis (2,371,400)*	St. Louis University			
	Washington University			

Area centers

Location	Institution	Type		Funding
Kansas City (1,301,600)* (serves 38 counties)	Western Missouri Area Health Education Center	Comprehensive	University of Missouri, Kansas City	BHM, University of Missouri, other ($9,122,700)

Other Carnegie Council suggested centers

MONTANA

Health science centers

Area centers

Institution	Type	
[Included in Washington, Alaska, Montana, Idaho, Program, Inc.—see Washington]	Area health education system	University of Washington School of Medicine

Carnegie Council suggested centers

NEBRASKA

Health science centers

Omaha (575,100)*	Creighton University
	University of Nebraska

Area centers

(continued on next page)

Table A-6 (continued)

State and city	Institution	Type of center	Health science center affiliation	Source and amount of funding, 1972-75
NEBRASKA (continued)				
Carnegie Council suggested centers				
North Platte (19,447)	[fully developed center suggested]	Area health education center		
Grand Island (31,269)	[suggestion repeated]	Area health education center		
Lincoln (182,200)*	[fully developed center suggested]	Area health education center		
NEVADA				
Health science centers				
Reno (142,700)*	University of Nevada, Reno			
Area centers				
none				
Carnegie Council suggested centers				
Las Vegas (319,600)*	[suggestion repeated]	Area health education center		
NEW HAMPSHIRE				
Health science centers				
Hanover (6,147)	Dartmouth Medical School			
Area centers				
none				
Carnegie Council suggested centers				
Berlin (15,256)	[suggestion repeated]	Area health education center		
Manchester (238,500)*	[suggestion repeated]	Area health education center		

NEW JERSEY

Health science centers

Newark (2,019,200)*	New Jersey College of Medicine		
New Brunswick (590,200)*	Rutgers Medical School		

Clinical training centers

Paterson (456,200)*			New Jersey College of Medicine
Hackensack (35,911)			New Jersey College of Medicine
Jersey City (583,000)*			New Jersey College of Medicine
Mountainside (7,520)			Columbia University

Area centers

Carnegie Council suggested centers

Trenton (319,000)*	[suggestion repeated]	Area health education center	
Camden (102,551)	[suggestion repeated]	Area health education center	
Atlantic City (190,000)*	[suggestion repeated]	Area health education center	

NEW MEXICO

Health science centers

Albuquerque (378,900)*	University of New Mexico		

Area centers

Albuquerque (378,900)* (serves Navajo Indian reservations in New Mexico and Arizona)	University of New Mexico Area Health Education Center	Comprehensive	University of New Mexico	BHM ($3,637,100)
Gallup (13,779)	University of New Mexico Area Health Education Center	Comprehensive	University of New Mexico	

Carnegie Council suggested centers

Roswell (33,908)	[suggestion repeated]	Area health education center	

(continued on next page)

Table A-6 (continued)

State and city	Institution	Type of center	Health science center affiliation	Source and amount of funding, 1972-75
NEW YORK				
Health science centers				
Buffalo (1,330,700)*	State University of New York			
Rochester (966,400)*	University of Rochester			
Syracuse (645,800)*	State University of New York			
Albany (799,400)*	Albany Medical College			
Brooklyn (9,634,400)*	State University of New York			
New York City (9,634,400)*	Cornell University Medical College			
	Albert Einstein College of Medicine			
	Columbia University			
	Mt. Sinai School of Medicine			
	New York Medical College			
	New York University			
Stony Brook (2,620,700)*	State University of New York			
Clinical training centers				
Manhasset (8,541)	Mary Bassett Hospital		Cornell University	
Area centers				
Cooperstown	Mary Bassett Hospital		Columbia University	Private (amount unavailable)
Jamaica (9,634,400)*	Allied Health Science Consortium of Greater Queens	Clinical education and educational development	City University of New York	HEW ($393,500)
Stony Brook (2,620,700)*	The Health Sciences Center[b]	Comprehensive	State University of New York, Stony Brook	State (amount not indicated)

Binghamton	[fully developed center suggested]			
Utica	[fully developed center suggested]			

NORTH CAROLINA

Health science centers

Winston-Salem (759,500)*	Bowman-Gray School of Medicine			
Durham (462,300)*	Duke University			
Chapel Hill (462,300)*	University of North Carolina			

Health science center in developing stage

Greenville (29,063)	East Carolina University School of Medicine (not recommended by Carnegie Council)			

Area centers

(Chapel Hill)	Area Health Education Centers Program of North Carolina, Inc.	Comprehensive	University of North Carolina, Chapel Hill	BHM, state, local ($22,667,000)
Asheville (166,300)*	Area Health Education Centers Program of North Carolina, Inc.	Comprehensive	University of North Carolina, Chapel Hill	
Northwest Planning Area	Area Health Education Centers Program of North Carolina, Inc.	Comprehensive	University of North Carolina, Chapel Hill	
Charlotte (589,300)*	Area Health Education Centers Program of North Carolina, Inc.	Comprehensive	University of North Carolina, Chapel Hill	
Greensboro (759,500)*	Area Health Education Centers Program of North Carolina, Inc.	Comprehensive	University of North Carolina, Chapel Hill	
Raleigh (462,300)*	Area Health Education Centers Program of North Carolina, Inc.	Comprehensive	University of North Carolina, Chapel Hill	
Fayetteville (223,100)*	Area Health Education Centers Program of North Carolina, Inc.	Comprehensive	University of North Carolina, Chapel Hill	

(continued on next page)

Table A-6 (*continued*)

State and city	Institution	Type of center	Health science center affiliation	Source and amount of funding, 1972-75
NORTH CAROLINA (*continued*)				
Area centers (*continued*)				
Greenville (29,063)	Area Health Education Centers Program of North Carolina, Inc.	Comprehensive	University of North Carolina, Chapel Hill	
Wilmington (126,900)*	Area Health Education Centers Program of North Carolina, Inc.	Comprehensive	University of North Carolina, Chapel Hill	
Health Planning Area L	Area Health Education Centers Program of North Carolina, Inc.	Comprehensive	University of North Carolina, Chapel Hill	
Other Carnegie Council suggested centers				
none				
NORTH DAKOTA				
Health science centers				
Grand Forks (39,008)	University of North Dakota			
Area centers				
(Grand Forks)	University of North Dakota School of Medicine AHEC	Clinical education and educational development	University of North Dakota	BHM ($2,052,000)
Minot (32,290)	University of North Dakota School of Medicine AHEC	Clinical education and educational development	University of North Dakota	
Bismark (34,703)	University of North Dakota School of Medicine AHEC	Clinical education and educational development	University of North Dakota	
Grand Forks (39,008)	University of North Dakota School of Medicine AHEC	Clinical education and educational development	University of North Dakota	

Fargo (125,600)*	University of North Dakota School of Medicine AHEC	Clinical education and educational development	University of North Dakota	

Other Carnegie Council suggested centers

OHIO

Health science centers

Cincinnati (1,375,800)*	University of Cincinnati			
Columbus (1,067,000)*	Ohio State University			
Toledo (781,000)*	Medical College of Ohio			
Cleveland (1,984,100)*	Case Western Reserve University			

Health science centers in developing stage

Kent (671,300)*	Northeastern Ohio Universities College of Medicine (not recommended by Carnegie Council)			
Dayton (844,800)*	Wright University (not recommended by Carnegie Council)			

Area centers

Cincinnati	The Health Education Alliance through the University of Cincinnati, Inc. (HEALTH–UC)	Comprehensive	University of Cincinnati	RMP, other ($123,000)

Other Carnegie Council suggested centers

Lima (210,800)*	[suggestion repeated]	Area health education center		
Mansfield (131,200)*	[suggestion repeated]	Area health education center		
Youngstown-Warren (542,900)	[suggestion repeated]	Area health education center		

(continued on next page)

Table A-6 (continued)

State and city	Institution	Type of center	Health science center affiliation	Source and amount of funding, 1972-75
OKLAHOMA				
Health science centers				
Oklahoma City (766,200)*	University of Oklahoma			
Tulsa (576,100)*	Oklahoma College of Osteo-pathic Medicine and Surgery			
Clinical training center				
Tulsa (576,100)*			University of Oklahoma School of Medicine	
Area centers				
none				
Carnegie Council suggested centers				
Enid (44,008)	[fully developed center suggested]			
Lawton (105,400)*	[fully developed center suggested]			
OREGON				
Health science centers				
Portland (1,079,700)*	University of Oregon			
Area centers				
none				
Carnegie Council suggested centers				
Eugene (236,600)*	[suggestion repeated]	Area health education center		
Medford (27,950)	[suggestion repeated]	Area health education center		

PENNSYLVANIA

Health science centers

Pittsburgh (2,333,600)* — University of Pittsburgh

Hershey (425,500)* — Pennsylvania State University

Philadelphia (4,809,900)* — Hahneman Medical College
Jefferson Medical College
The Medical College of Pennsylvania
Temple University
University of Pennsylvania
Philadelphia College of Osteopathic Medicine

Area centers

Carnegie Council suggested centers

Erie (273,700)* — [fully developed center suggested]

Altoona (135,600)* — [suggestion repeated] — Area health education center

Scranton/Wilkes-Barre/Hazleton (633,100)* — [suggestion repeated]

York (345,900)* — [suggestion repeated]

Allentown (616,600)* — [fully developed center suggested]

RHODE ISLAND

Health science centers

Providence (854,400)* — Brown University

Area centers

Carnegie Council suggested centers

(continued on next page)

Table A-6 (*continued*)

State and city	Institution	Type of center	Health science center affiliation	Source and amount of funding, 1972-75
SOUTH CAROLINA				
Health science centers				
Charleston (362,000)*	Medical University of South Carolina			
Health science center in developing stage				
Columbia (360,800)*	University of South Carolina			
Area centers				
(Charleston)	Medical University of South Carolina Area Health Education Centers	Comprehensive	Medical University of South Carolina	BHM, state, Robert Wood Johnson Foundation ($27,192,600)
Greenville (522,200)*	Medical University of South Carolina AHEC	Comprehensive	Medical University of South Carolina	
Spartanburg (522,200)*	Medical University of South Carolina AHEC	Comprehensive	Medical University of South Carolina	
Columbia (360,800)*	Medical University of South Carolina AHEC	Comprehensive	Medical University of South Carolina	
Florence (25,997)	Medical University of South Carolina AHEC	Comprehensive	Medical University of South Carolina	
Charleston (362,000)*	Medical University of South Carolina AHEC	Comprehensive	Medical University of South Carolina	
Other Carnegie Council suggested centers				
none				
SOUTH DAKOTA				
Health science centers				
Vermillion (9,128)	University of South Dakota			

(continued on next page)

Center	Institution	Coordinating center	Activities	Funding
Clinical training centers				
Yankton (11,919)	University of South Dakota			
Sioux Falls (98,400)*	University of South Dakota			
Area centers				
none				
Carnegie Council suggested centers				
Rapid City (43,836)	[fully developed center suggested]			
TENNESSEE				
Health science centers				
Memphis (853,100)*	University of Tennessee			
Nashville (744,600)*	Meharry Medical College			
	Vanderbilt University			
Health science center in developing stage				
Johnson City (391,700)*	East Tennessee State University (not recommended by Carnegie Council)			
Area centers				
Chattanooga (390,300)* (serves 10 counties in Tennessee and 3 counties in Georgia)	Southeast Tennessee Area Health Education Center	University of Tennessee Center for Health Sciences, Knoxville	Clinical education and educational development	RMP, University of Tennessee, other ($294,000)
Other Carnegie Council suggested centers				
Knoxville (427,700)*	[fully developed center suggested]			
TEXAS				
Health science centers				
Lubbock (194,500)*	Texas Technological University			
Dallas (2,498,500)*	University of Texas Southwestern			

State and city	Institution	Type of center	Health science center affiliation	Source and amount of funding, 1972-75
TEXAS (continued)				
Health science centers (continued)				
Fort Worth (2,498,500)*	Texas College of Osteopathic Medicine			
San Antonio (979,900)*	University of Texas Medical School			
Houston (2,222,700)*	Baylor University			
	University of Texas Medical School			
Galveston (179,100)*	University of Texas Medical Branch			
Health science center in developing stage				
College Station (67,900)*	Texas A&M University and Baylor College of Medicine (not recommended by Carnegie Council)			
Clinical training centers				
El Paso (410,000)*			Texas Technological University	Texas Technological University
Amarillo (150,200)*			Texas Technological University	Texas Technological University
Big Spring (28,735)			Texas Technological University	Texas Technological University
Area centers				
(Galveston)	University of Texas Allied Health Education Center Program—Medical Branch at Galveston	Comprehensive	University of Texas Medical Branch, Galveston	BHM ($2,996,700)
Temple (33,431)	University of Texas Allied Health Education Center Program—Medical Branch at	Comprehensive	University of Texas Medical Branch, Galveston	

Laredo (78,100)*	University of Texas Allied Health Education Center Program—Medical Branch at Galveston	Comprehensive	University of Texas Medical Branch, Galveston
Corpus Christi (295,100)*	University of Texas Allied Health Education Center Program—Medical Branch at Galveston	Comprehensive	University of Texas Medical Branch, Galveston
Edinburg (17,163)	University of Texas Allied Health Education Center Program—Medical Branch at Galveston	Comprehensive	University of Texas Medical Branch, Galveston

Other Carnegie Council suggested centers

| Beaumont (344,600)* | [suggestion repeated] | Area health education center | |

UTAH

Health science centers

| Salt Lake City (765,500)* | University of Utah | | |

Area centers

Carnegie Council suggested centers

| Cedar City (8,946) | [suggestion repeated] | Area health education center | |

VERMONT

Health science centers

| Burlington (38,633) | University of Vermont | | |

Area centers

Carnegie Council suggested centers

| Rutland (19,293) | [suggestion repeated] | Area health education center | |

(continued on next page)

Table A-6 (continued)

State and city	Institution	Type of center	Health science center affiliation	Source and amount of funding, 1972-75
VIRGINIA				
Health science centers				
Charlottesville (38,880)	University of Virginia			
Richmond (569,500)*	Medical College of Virginia			
Norfolk/Portsmouth (766,000)*	Eastern Virginia Medical School (developing—operational)			
Area centers				
none				
Carnegie Council suggested centers				
Roanoke (212,200)*	[suggestion repeated]	Area health education center		
WASHINGTON				
Health science centers				
Seattle (1,396,400)*	University of Washington School of Medicine			
Area centers				
Seattle (1,396,400)*	Washington, Alaska, Montana, Idaho Program, Inc.	Comprehensive	University of Washington School of Medicine	NIH, HEW, states ($1,115,100)
Other Carnegie Council suggested centers				
none				
WEST VIRGINIA				
Health science centers				
Morgantown (29,431)	West Virginia University			
Lewisburg (2,407)	West Virginia School of Osteopathic Medicine			

Health science center in developing stage				
Huntington (290,400)*	Marshall University (not recommended by Carnegie Council)			
Area centers				
Charleston (253,700)* (serves 6 counties)	WVU-CAMC Area Health Education Center	Comprehensive	West Virginia University School of Medicine	BHM, state, other ($8,425,000)
Other Carnegie Council suggested centers				
Parkersburg (150,000)*	[suggestion repeated]	Area health education center		
WISCONSIN				
Health science centers				
Madison (303,000)*	University of Wisconsin			
Milwaukee (1,415,400)*	Medical College of Wisconsin			
Clinical training centers				
Marshfield (15,619)	Gunderson Clinic		University of Wisconsin Medical School	
La Crosse (83,300)*	Marshfield Clinic		University of Wisconsin Medical School	
Milwaukee (1,415,400)*	Mt. Sinai Clinic		University of Wisconsin Medical School	
Area centers				
none				
Carnegie Council suggested centers				
Eau Claire (123,700)*	[suggestion repeated]			
Green Bay (166,600)*	[suggestion repeated]			
WYOMING				
Health science centers				
none				
Area centers				
none				

(continued on next page)

Table A-6 (*continued*)

State and city	Institution	Type of center	Health science center affiliation	Source and amount of funding, 1972-75
WYOMING (*continued*)				
Carnegie Council suggested centers				
Caspar (39,361)	[suggestion repeated]	Area health education center		
Cheyenne	[fully developed center suggested]			

*Estimated population of Standard Metropolitan Statistical Areas, 1974.

+Population of Standard Metropolitan Statistical Area, 1970.

aMaryland has recently passed legislation to develop a system of area health education centers to be affiliated with the University of Maryland School of Medicine.

bThe Pagan Associates report indicates that the Stony Brook center serves New York State, but its activities appear to be largely centered on Long Island.

VA = Veterans Administration
RMP = Regional Medical Program
BHM = Bureau of Health Manpower
NIMH = National Institutes of Mental Health
HEW = U.S. Department of Health, Education and Welfare
PHS = Public Health Service

Source: "Medical Education in the United States, 1974-1975"; Pagan Associates (1975); and other miscellaneous sources.

Table A-7. State expenditures on educational general purpose programs
of medical schools, per $1,000,000 personal income, 1965-67 (average of
two years) and 1973-74 (states arranged by rank in 1973-74)

State	1965-67	Rank	1973-74	Rank	Changes in rank
United States	$ 253		$ 479		
Vermont	1,118	2	1,647	1	+1
Texas	304	17	1,144	2	+15
Arizona	44	37	931	3	+34
Kansas	234	29	913	4	+25
South Carolina	433	8	877	5	+3
Alabama	382	11	827	6	+5
West Virginia	559	5	782	7	−2
Kentucky	731	3	750	8	−5
Oregon	343	13	723	9	+4
Utah	1,242	1	654	10	−9
Michigan	344	12	652	11	+1
Mississippi	394	10	624	12	−2
Washington	306	16	582	13	+3
Louisiana	525	6	565	14	−8
Colorado	249	24	543	15	+8
Nebraska	292	19	541	16	+3
New Mexico	10	40	534	17	+23
Indiana	294	18	503	18	0
North Carolina	164	34	499	19	+15
Illinois	124	35	492	20	+15
Georgia	235	28	490	21	+7
Iowa	718	4	447	22	−18
Wisconsin	275	20	432	23	−3
New York	248	25	428	24	+1
New Jersey	70	36	424	25	+11
Arkansas	482	7	409	26	−19
Florida	230	30	396	27	+3
Hawaii	n.a.		393	28	n.a.
Pennsylvania	257	22	389	29	−7
California	238	27	386	30	−3
Ohio	259	21	382	31	−10
Connecticut	11	39	378	32	+7

(continued on next page)

Table A-7 *(continued)*

State	1965-67	Rank	1973-74	Rank	Changes in rank
Minnesota	$ 395	9	$ 354	33	−24
Oklahoma	228	32	344	34	−2
North Dakota	331	14	340	35	−21
Missouri	230	31	324	36	−5
Tennessee	330	15	309	37	−22
South Dakota	251	23	261	38	−15
Maryland	165	33	230	39	−6
Nevada	16	38	180	40	−2
Massachusetts	10	41	178	41	0
Virginia	242	26	159	42	−16
Rhode Island	9	43	85	43	0
New Hampshire	9	42	72	44	−2

Sources: Fein and Weber (1971, pp. 140-143) and "State Roles in Financing Medical Education" (1976, p. 207). Data for additional states on Map 5 obtained from the New England Board of Higher Education and the Western Interstate Commission on Higher Education.

Table A-8. State financial support of medical and dental education in private schools, 1974-75

State	Type of support	
	Medical education	Dental education
Alabama	Support through SREB	Support through SREB
Alaska	Support through WICHE	Support through WICHE
Arizona	Support through WICHE	Support through WICHE
Arkansas	No private school—no program	Support through SREB
California	Capitation payments for enrollment increases	No program
	Support for clinical training of FMGs	
Colorado	No private school—no program	No private school—no program
Connecticut	No program	No private school—no program
Delaware	Support for 20 students at Jefferson Medical College (Penna.)	No dental school—no program
Florida	Capitation payments for Florida residents at University of Miami School of Medicine	No private school—no program
	Support through SREB	

Table A-8

	Type of support	
State	*Medical education*	*Dental education*
Georgia	Capitation payments for Emory University School of Medicine through SREB	No program
Hawaii	No private school—no program	No dental school—no program
Idaho	Support through WICHE	Support through WICHE
Illinois	Grants for increased enrollment of Illinois residents	Grants for increased enrollment of Illinois residents
Indiana	No private school—no program	No private school—no program
Iowa	Support for Iowa residents enrolled in Des Moines College of Osteopathic Medicine and Surgery	No private school—no program
Kansas	No private school—no program	No private school—no program
Kentucky	No private school[a]—no program	No private school[a]—no program
Louisiana	Capitation payments for Louisiana residents at Tulane University School of Medicine Support through SREB	Support through SREB
Maine	Support through NEBHE	Support through NEBHE
Maryland	Capitation payments for Johns Hopkins University School of Medicine, but not effective until 1976-77 Support through SREB	Support through SREB
Massachusetts	Scholarship program Support through NEBHE	Scholarship program
Michigan	No private school—no program	Contracts for dental school services for Michigan residents
Minnesota	Capitation payments for Minnesota residents at Mayo Medical School Medical student loan program—obligation to practice in rural community for 3 years	No private school—no program
Mississippi	Support through SREB	Support through SREB
Missouri	No program	No program
Montana	Support through WICHE	Support through WICHE
Nebraska	No program	No program
Nevada	Support through WICHE	Support through WICHE
New Hampshire	Support for small number of state residents at Dartmouth Medical School	No dental school—no program

(continued on next page)

Table A-8 *(continued)*

| State | Type of support | |
	Medical education	Dental education
New Jersey	No private school—no program	No program
New Mexico	Support through WICHE	Support through WICHE; and subsidies for dental students in states outside WICHE
New York	Scholarship program; higher awards for limited number of students agreeing to serve in underserved areas Capitation payments for private medical schools Capitation payments for enrollment increases	Scholarship program Capitation payments for enrollment increases
North Carolina	Grants to private schools for education of North Carolina residents Loan program Support through SREB	Loan program Support through SREB
North Dakota	Contract with Mayo Medical School for up to 5 3rd-year North Dakota medical students[b]	No dental school—no program
Ohio	Capitation payments for Case Western Reserve University School of Medicine	Capitation payments for Case Western Reserve University School of Dentistry
Oklahoma	No private school—no program	No private school—no program
Oregon	No private school—no program	No private school—no program
Pennsylvania	Private medical schools receive state funds through state program of support for 12 private institutions	Private dental schools receive state funds through state program of support for 12 private institutions
Rhode Island	Grants to Brown University Program in Medical Science Support through NEBHE	No dental school—no program
South Carolina	Scholarships (forgiveness grants for practice in rural areas)	Scholarships (forgiveness grants for practice in rural areas)
South Dakota	Loans for completion of training outside state (repayment deferred for each year of practice in South Dakota)	No dental school—no program
Tennessee	Capitation payments to private schools for increasing enrollment of state residents Loan-scholarship program for medical students who intend to practice in shortage area of state Support through SREB	Support through SREB

Table A-8

	Type of support	
State	Medical education	Dental education
Texas	Contracts with Baylor University for medical training of Texas residents	Contracts with Baylor University for dental training of Texas residents
	Contracts with Texas College of Osteopathic Medicine for Texas undergraduate medical students	
Utah	No private school—no program	No dental school—no program
Vermont	No private school—no program	No dental school—no program
Virginia	Capitation payments to Eastern Virginia Medical School	Support through SREB
	Support through SREB	
Washington	No private school—no program	No private school—no program
West Virginia	No private school—no program	No private school—no program
Wisconsin	Grants for Medical College of Wisconsin	Contracts to provide dental education to state residents at Marquette University School of Dentistry
Wyoming	Support through WICHE	Support through WICHE

[a]The University of Louisville is now state supported.

[b]Similar contract with University of Minnesota Medical School for 35 students.

Sources: "State Roles in Financing Medical Education" (1976); Millard (1975); and other sources. It should be noted that scholarships and loans are available for medical and dental students under general student aid programs in some of the states, but we have included in this table only scholarship and loan programs specifically intended for health professions students.

NEBHE = New England Board of Higher Education
SREB = Southern Regional Education Board
WICHE = Western Interstate Commission for Higher Education

Appendix B

Projections of Physician Supply

Low Projection

1. The size of future entering classes was estimated by studying the planned increases in the 114 medical schools now in operation, on the basis of their actual first-year enrollment in 1974-75 and their projected enrollment in 1975-76 and 1977-78, as reported in Association of American Medical Colleges (1976a). All available information on maximum planned size of entering classes was also used. A small adjustment was made to allow for enrollment increases that might occur but that were not indicated by these sources of information. An estimate of future first-year enrollment in schools of osteopathy was based on a study of changes in their first-year enrollment in recent years. No allowance was made for enrollment in schools not yet in operation. The number of entrants rises to 17,300 in 1981-82 and then levels off.
2. The size of future graduating classes was estimated by analyzing ratios of numbers of graduates to numbers of entrants four years earlier in recent years. Because of the rising proportion of students who have been graduating under three-year programs, this ratio has risen above one in the last few years. We have assumed that the proportion of students graduating in three years will not rise significantly in the future and that the ratio of the number of graduates to the number

of entrants four years earlier will gradually fall back to .96 as the number of entrants levels off.

3. We have assumed that the net increase in the number of active FMGs in the United States will decline to 2,000 by 1979-80, and that this number will consist of visiting FMGs entering for postgraduate training on temporary visas. From that point on we have assumed no net increase in the number of active FMGs (each annual group of visiting scholars will be replaced by an equal number, but there will be no net addition).

4. Attrition rates (retirements and deaths) have been adapted from those used in U.S. Public Health Service (1974).

High Projection

1. We have added first-year enrollment in 13 developing schools, on the assumption that they will gradually reach their planned maximum first-year enrollment by 1980-81, to first-year enrollment as projected in the low projection. This is to be interpreted as an assumption for estimating purposes, not as an endorsement of all 13 of these schools (see Section 6). This could actually turn out to be a conservative assumption, because the number of developing schools may continue to increase if vigorous measures are not taken to stop the trend toward adding new schools. On the basis of this high projection, the number of entrants rises to 18,210 in 1981-82 and then levels off.

2. The method used in projecting the number of graduates was the same as in connection with the low projection.

3. We have assumed that the net increase in the number of FMGs will decline more slowly than under the low projection. From 1986-87 on, 2,000 FMGs will enter each year on a visiting-scholar basis, but there will be no net increase in the number of active FMGs.

4. The method of estimating attrition was the same as in connection with the low projection.

References

American Association of Dental Schools. *Admission Requirements of U.S. and Canadian Dental Schools, 1976-77.* Washington, D.C., 1975a.

American Association of Dental Schools. *Bulletin of Dental Education,* October 1975b, *8* (10).

American Dental Association. *Annual Report, 1975-76: Dental Education Supplement #4: Financial Report, Fiscal Year Ending June 30, 1975.* Chicago, n.d.

American Dental Association, in cooperation with American Association of Dental Schools. *Annual Report, Dental Education: 1975-76.* Chicago, 1975.

American Medical Association. *Physician Distribution and Medical Licensure in the U.S., 1974.* Chicago, 1975.

Association of American Medical Colleges. *Undergraduate Medical Education: Elements—Objectives—Costs.* Report of the Committee on the Financing of Medical Education. Washington, D.C., 1973.

Association of American Medical Colleges. *Medical School Admission Requirements, 1975-76.* Washington, D.C., 1974.

Association of American Medical Colleges. *Medical School Admission Requirements, 1977-78.* Washington, D.C., 1976a.

Association of American Medical Colleges. *Weekly Report,* #76-15, Apr. 12, 1976b.

Beall, J. G., Jr. Statement in *Health Manpower Legislation, 1975.* Part 2, pp. 927-944. Washington, D.C.: U.S. Government Printing Office, 1976. (Full citation under Kennedy, E. M.)

Bennett, I., and Cooper, J. A. D. Statement in *Health Manpower Legislation, 1975.* Part 4, pp. 2053-2065. Washington, D.C.: U.S. Government Printing Office, 1976. (Full citation under Kennedy, E. M.)

Blumberg, M. S. *Trends and Projections of Physicians in the United States, 1967-2002.* Berkeley, Calif.: Carnegie Commission on Higher Education, 1971.

Boffey, P. M. "Medical Schools Told They Face U.S. Cutbacks." *Chronicle of Higher Education,* Nov. 12, 1973.

Bunker, J. P. "Surgical Manpower." *New England Journal of Medicine,* Jan. 15, 1970, *282* (3).

Carnegie Commission on Higher Education. *Higher Education and the Nation's Health: Policies for Medical and Dental Education.* New York: McGraw-Hill, 1970.

Carnegie Commission on Higher Education. *The More Effective Use of Resources: An Imperative for Higher Education.* New York: McGraw-Hill, 1972.

Carnegie Council on Higher Education. *Low or No Tuition: The Feasibility of a National Policy for the First Two Years of College.* San Francisco: Jossey-Bass, 1975a.

Carnegie Council on Higher Education. *The Federal Role in Postsecondary Education: Unfinished Business, 1975-1980.* San Francisco: Jossey-Bass, 1975b.

Carnegie Foundation for the Advancement of Teaching. *The States and Higher Education: A Proud Past and a Vital Future.* San Francisco: Jossey-Bass, 1976.

Comptroller General of the United States. *Congressional Objectives of Federal Loans and Scholarships to Health Professions Students Not Being Met.* Washington, D.C.: U.S. Government Printing Office, 1974.

Cooper, J. A. D. "Education for the Health Professions in the Soviet Union." *Journal of Medical Education,* May 1971, *46* (5), 412-418.

Cooper, J. A. D. Statement in *Health Manpower Programs.* Washington, D.C., 1975, pp. 465-479. (Full citation under Weinberger, C. W.)

Cooper, T. Statement in *Health Manpower Legislation, 1975.* Part 2, pp. 945-1050. Washington, D.C., 1976. (Full citation under Kennedy, E. M.)

"The Dance of Legislation: A Case History." *Technology Review,* June 1974.

"Dartmouth to Drop Physician Assistants Program." *Chronicle of Higher Education,* Apr. 7, 1975.

Dewey, D. *Where the Doctors Have Gone: The Changing Distribution of Private Practice Physicians in the Chicago Metropolitan Area, 1950-1970.* Chicago: Illinois Regional Medical Program, 1973.

"Doctors Are Slow to Accept Non-Doctor Assistants." *New York Times,* May 11, 1976.

Economic Report of the President, 1976. Washington, D.C.: U.S. Government Printing Office, 1976.

Education Commission of the States. *Higher Education in the States.* Denver, Colo., annual.

Enthoven, A. C. "Can We Control the Cost of Health Care?". Reprint Series, Graduate School of Business, Stanford University, No. 214. Stanford, Calif., 1976.

Estes, E. H., Jr., and Howard, D. R. "Potential for New Classes of Personnel: Experiences of the Duke Physician's Assistant Program." *Journal of Medical Education,* March 1970, *45,* 149-155.

Fein, R. *The Doctor Shortage: An Economic Diagnosis.* Washington, D.C.: The Brookings Institution, 1967.

Fein, R., and Weber, G. I. *Financing Medical Education: An Analysis of Alternative Policies and Mechanisms.* New York: McGraw-Hill, 1971.

Feldstein, M. "The Rising Price of Physicians' Services." *Review of Economics and Statistics*, May 1970, *52* (2), 121-133.

Fuchs, V. R. *Who Shall Live? Health, Economics, and Social Choice.* New York: Basic Books, 1974.

Garrard, J., and Weber, R. "Comparison of Three- and Four-Year Medical School Graduates." *Journal of Medical Education*, June 1974, *49* (6), 547-553.

"Graduates of Foreign Medical Schools in the United States: A Challenge to Medical Education." *Journal of Medical Education*, August 1974, *49* (8), 809-822.

Held, P. J., and Reinhardt, U. E. "Health Manpower Policy in a Market Context." Paper presented at annual meeting of American Economic Association, Dallas, Texas, Dec. 28-30, 1975 (not included in published proceedings).

"HEW Awarded 895 PHS Scholarships." *Higher Education Daily*, July 1, 1976.

"HEW Mails Public Health Service Scholarship Forms." *Higher Education Daily*, Oct. 16, 1975.

Hicks, N. "Health Corps Aids Doctors and Communities." *New York Times*, June 18, 1974.

Holden, W. D., and others. Statement in *Health Manpower Legislation, 1975.* Part 3, pp. 1423-1436. Washington, D.C., 1976. (Full citation under Kennedy, E. M.)

Hollister, R., Kramer, B., and Bellin, S. *Neighborhood Health Centers.* Lexington, Mass.: D. C. Heath Co., 1974.

Illich, I. *Medical Nemesis: The Expropriation of Health.* New York: Pantheon Books, 1976.

Josiah Macy, Jr. Foundation. *Report of the Commission on Physicians for the Future.* New York (advance copy), 1976.

Kennedy, E. M. Statement in *Health Manpower Legislation, 1975.* Hearings Before the Subcommittee on Health, Committee on Labor and Public Welfare, U.S. Senate, 94th Cong., 1st Sess., Part 2, pp. 923-926. Washington, D.C., 1976.

Klarman, H. E. *The Economics of Health.* New York: Columbia University Press, 1965.

Lawrence, D., Wilson, W., and Castle, H. "Employment of MEDEX Graduates and Trainees: Five-Year Progress Report for the United States." *Journal of the American Medical Association*, Oct. 13, 1975, *234* (2), 174-177.

Lee, P. R. Statement in *Health Manpower Programs*, pp. 371-437. Washington, D.C., 1975. (Full citation under Weinberger, C. W.)

Lee, P. R. Statement in *Health Manpower Legislation, 1975.* Part 3, pp. 1685-1801. Washington, D.C., 1976. (Full citation under Kennedy, E. M.)

Lee, P. R., and others. *Primary Care in a Specialized World: The Failure of Health Manpower Policies.* Forthcoming, 1976.

Lewis, C. E. "Variations in the Incidence of Surgery." *New England Journal of Medicine*, 1969, *281* (16), 880-884.

"Medical Center Eyed for City." *Cumberland, Md. Times,* Mar. 14, 1976.

"Medical Course of 3 Years Tried." *New York Times,* Oct. 21, 1973.

"Medical Education in the United States, 1970-1971." *Journal of the American Medical Association,* Nov. 22, 1971, *218* (8), 1199-1316.

"Medical Education in the United States, 1973-1974." 74th Annual Report. *Journal of the American Medical Association,* Supplement. January 1975, *231,* 1-139.

"Medical Education in the United States, 1974-75." 75th Annual Report. *Journal of the American Medical Association,* Dec. 29, 1975, *234* (13), 1325-1432.

"Medical School Admissions: A Glimpse at the Future by Looking Back." *Journal of Medical Education,* September 1975, *50* (9), 912-914.

"Medical School Enrollment, 1971-72 to 1975-76." *Journal of Medical Education,* February 1976, *51* (2), 144-146.

Miike, L. H., and Ross, R. J. "Area Health Education Centers: What Are They and Where Are They Going?". *Journal of Medical Education,* March 1975, *50* (3), 242-251.

Millard, R. M. "The States and Private Higher Education." *Higher Education in the States,* 1975, *5* (1), 1-24.

Mueller, M. S., and Gibson, R. M. "National Health Expenditures, Fiscal Year 1975." *Social Security Bulletin,* February 1976, *39* (2), 3-20, 48.

Mueller, M. S., and Piro, P. A. "Private Health Insurance in 1974: A Review of Coverage, Enrollment, and Financial Experience." *Social Security Bulletin,* March 1976, *39* (3), 3-20.

National Academy of Sciences, Institute of Medicine. *Costs of Education in the Health Professions.* Washington, D.C., 1974.

Nesbitt, T. E., and Ruhe, C. H. W. Statement in *Health Manpower Programs,* pp. 508-524. Washington, D.C., 1975. (Full citation under Weinberger, C. W.)

Nesbitt, T. E., Ruhe, C. H. W., and Peterson, H. Statement in *Health Manpower Legislation, 1975.* Part 4, pp. 1996-2053. Washington, D.C., 1976. (Full citation under Kennedy, E. M.)

Pagan, C. E., Associates, Inc. *Area Health Education Centers: A Directory of Federal, State, Local and Private Decentralized Health Professional Education Programs.* Report prepared for Bureau of Health Manpower. Bethesda, Md., 1975.

Page, R. G. "The Three-Year Medical Curriculum." *Journal of the American Medical Association,* Aug. 10, 1970, *213* (6), 1012-1015.

Page, R. G., and Boulger, J. G. "An Assessment of the Three-Year Medical Curriculum." *Journal of Medical Education,* February 1976, *51* (2), 125-126.

"Physician's Aide Review Bodies Merge." *Higher Education Daily,* Dec. 16, 1975.

Redig, D. F. Statement in *Health Manpower Programs,* pp. 606-611. Washington, D.C., 1975. (Full citation under Weinberger, C. W.)

Rovin, S. *A Curriculum for Primary Care Dentistry.* Unpublished paper, School of Dentistry, University of Washington, 1976.

"Service by Health Students." *Chronicle of Higher Education,* July 21, 1975.

Shira, R. B. Statement in *Health Manpower Legislation, 1975.* Part 4, pp. 2065-2087. Washington, D.C., 1976. (Full citation under Kennedy, E. M.)

Smythe, C. McC. "New Resources for Medical Education: Start-Up Expenditures in 22 New Medical Schools." *Journal of Medical Education,* September 1972, *47* (9), 690-701.

Spingarn, N. D. "Test This Week to Certify Physicians' Assistants for First Time." *Chronicle of Higher Education,* Dec. 10, 1973.

"State Funding for Targeted Programs in Graduate Medical Education." *Journal of Medical Education,* June 1974, *49* (6), 620-622.

"State Roles in Financing Medical Education." *Journal of Medical Education,* March 1976, *51* (3), 206-209.

Stevens, R. *American Medicine and the Public Interest.* New Haven and London: Yale University Press, 1971.

Stevens, R. Dissenting comment in Josiah Macy, Jr. Foundation. *Report of the Commission on Physicians for the Future.* New York (advance copy), 1976.

Stevens, R., and others. "Physician Migration Reexamined." *Science,* Oct. 31, 1975, *190,* 439-442.

Supplemental Appropriations for Fiscal Year 1976. Hearings Before Subcommittee of the Committee on Appropriations, U.S. House of Representatives. Washington, D.C., 1975.

Swanson, A. G. "Area Health Education Centers Versus an Area Health Education System." *Journal of Medical Education,* May 1972, *47* (5), 321-326.

U.S. Bureau of the Census. *Statistical Abstract of the United States.* Washington, D.C.: U.S. Government Printing Office, annual.

U.S. Department of Health, Education, and Welfare. *Area Health Education Centers.* DHEW Publication No. (HRA) 74-7. Washington, D.C.: U.S. Government Printing Office, 1973.

U.S. Department of Health, Education, and Welfare. *Current Estimates from the Health Interview Survey, United States—1974,* Vital and Health Statistics, Series 10. Washington, D.C.: U.S. Government Printing Office, 1975a.

U.S. Department of Health, Education, and Welfare. *Neighborhood Health Centers, Summary of Project Data No. 10.* Washington, D.C.: U.S. Government Printing Office, 1975b.

U.S. Department of Health, Education, and Welfare. *Proceedings of the National Conference, the Area Health Education Centers Program.* Asheville, North Carolina, April 25-27, 1975. DHEW Publication No. (HRA) 76-38. Washington, D.C.: U.S. Government Printing Office, 1976a.

U.S. Department of Health, Education, and Welfare. *Report of the President's Biomedical Research Panel.* Submitted to the President and the Congress of the United States. DHEW Publication No. (OS) 76-500. Washington, D.C.: U.S. Government Printing Office, 1976b.

U.S. Department of Health, Education, and Welfare. *Total Loss of Teeth in Adults.* Washington, D.C.: U.S. Government Printing Office, 1967.

U.S. House of Representatives, Subcommittee on Health, Committee on

Ways and Means. *Medicare-Medicaid Reimbursement Policies.* Social Security Studies Final Report Submitted by the Institute of Medicine, National Academy of Sciences. 95th Cong., 2d Sess. Washington, D.C.: U.S. Government Printing Office, 1976.

"U.S. Medical School Enrollment, 1970-71 Through 1974-75." *Journal of Medical Education.* March 1975, *50* (3), 303-306.

U.S. National Center of Health Statistics. *Health Resources Statistics.* Washington, D.C.: U.S. Government Printing Office, annual.

U.S. Office of Management and Budget. *Social Indicators, 1973.* Washington, D.C.: U.S. Government Printing Office, 1973.

U.S. Public Health Service. *The Supply of Health Manpower: 1970 Profiles and Projections to 1990.* Washington, D.C.: U.S. Government Printing Office, 1974.

U.S. Senate, Committee on Appropriations. *Second Supplemental Appropriation FY 1975.* Washington, D.C.: U.S. Government Printing Office, 1975.

U.S. Senate, Committee on Labor and Public Welfare. *Health Professions Educational Assistance Act of 1976.* Report No. 94-887. 94th Cong., 2d Sess. Washington, D.C.: U.S. Government Printing Office, 1976.

Watkins, B. T. "Dental Educators Ask for Criticism—and Get It." *Chronicle of Higher Education,* Mar. 31, 1975.

Wechsler, H., Williams, A. F., and Thum, D. "Dentistry in 1980—Predictions by Deans of Dental Schools." *Journal of Dental Education,* April 1972a, 14-15.

Wechsler, H., Williams, A., and Thum, D. "Maldistribution of Dental Manpower: A Cause for National Concern." *Journal of the American College of Dentists,* July 1972b, *39,* 151-160.

Weinberger, C. W. Statement in *Health Manpower Programs,* pp. 308-366. Subcommittee on Health and the Environment, Committee on Interstate and Foreign Commerce, U.S. House of Representatives, 94th Cong., 1st Sess. Washington, D.C., 1975.

Yett, D. E., and Sloan, F. A. "Migration Patterns of Recent Medical School Graduates." *Inquiry,* June 1974, 11 (2), 125-142.

"1,480 NHSC Scholarships Awarded in FY 75." *Higher Education Daily,* July 10, 1975.

Index